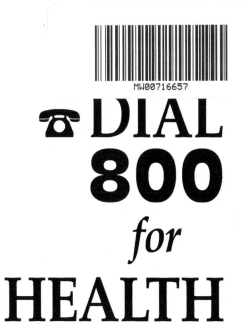

☎ DIAL
800
for
HEALTH

OTHER BOOKS FROM
THE PEOPLE'S MEDICAL SOCIETY

☎ DIAL 800 for HEALTH

Compiled and Tested by the People's Medical Society

≡People's Medical Society®

Allentown, Pennsylvania

The People's Medical Society is a nonprofit consumer health organization dedicated to the principles of better, more responsive and less expensive medical care. Organized in 1983, the People's Medical Society puts previously unavailable medical information into the hands of consumers so that they can make informed decisions about their own health care.

Membership in the People's Medical Society is $20 a year and includes a subscription to the *People's Medical Society Newsletter*. For information, write to the People's Medical Society, 462 Walnut Street, Allentown, PA 18102, or call 610-770-1670.

This and other People's Medical Society publications are available for quantity purchase at discount. Contact the People's Medical Society for details.

© 1993, 1997 by the People's Medical Society
Printed in the United States of America

Library of Congress Cataloging-in-Publication Data
Dial 800 for health / compiled and tested by the People's
   Medical Society.
    p. cm.
   Includes index.
   ISBN 1-882606-30-2
   1. Health education—Directories. 2. Health—Information
services—Directories. 3. Medical care—Information services—
Directories. 4. Preventive health services—Directories. 5. Toll-free
telephone calls—Directories. I. People's Medical Society (U.S.)
RA440.5.D49   1997
362.1'025'73—dc21   97-12305
                                                                          CIP
1 2 3 4 5 6 7 8 9 0
First printing, September 1997

CONTENTS

INTRODUCTION

The emerging consumer health movement has spawned an army of well-informed, proactive individuals who no longer limit their sources of health and medical information to their personal physicians. These empowered consumers now look to a wide array of professional and consumer-oriented organizations for vital medical and health-care information. No longer do consumers have limited access to cutting-edge data about specific conditions, medications or treatment options. A nationwide network of self-help and support groups has been formed around interests such as adoption services, organ transplants, substance abuse counseling and women's health.

In this book, the People's Medical Society has assembled more than 400 useful and important health-related organizations that offer toll-free telephone numbers for public use. You are bound to find the right organization to help you in your specific search for necessary health data. For example, *Dial 800 for Health* gives you access to agencies and organizations that can tell you about a medical condition, answer your questions about toxic substances, test your hearing over the phone or locate a local support group. And you don't need to leave your home to obtain any of this information. The only piece of equipment you need is your telephone.

With literally hundreds of groups to choose from, you're sure to find one that meets your particular needs and interests. And you won't spend a fortune making long-distance calls. Some groups listed in this directory are clearinghouses—services that can point you to an organization in or near your own community to help you directly. Others offer free information packets. Still others have answering machines so that you can leave your own message or request additional information. Many organizations also offer e-mail, and we've included those e-mail addresses that are available.

The majority of organizations listed in this book are nonprofit agencies, though a few are profit-making businesses. Much of the information is provided free; however, some organizations may charge a small service fee for material they provide. In addition, these organizations may offer publications for sale. But there is never a charge for the phone call.

Keeping up with all the new and important health-care information that emerges on a daily basis is difficult. But *Dial 800 for Health* is your entrée to vital medical and health information that was previously hard to find.

Use it for good health.

HOW TO USE THIS DIRECTORY

Dial 800 for Health is like having your own personal health-care researcher to provide you with the answers and information you need to make important health-care decisions. The table of contents alphabetically lists major headings such as adoption, cancer, health information and women's health. By turning directly to the page listed for a particular condition or service, you will find the organizations and agencies that can help you. Included for each organization are the name, address, toll-free telephone number, hours of operation and type of information or service provided.

The index and subject cross-reference found in the back of the book can help you to locate an agency or organization even if you can't find it listed in the table of contents. For example, if you want information on Crohn's disease and you didn't find it listed among the major headings, turn to the index and subject cross-reference and locate Crohn's disease, which then directs you to the section on digestive diseases.

Types of Toll-Free Numbers

This edition of *Dial 800 for Health* includes listings within the new *888* toll-free telephone exchange, which was added when the supply of toll-free *800* numbers was exhausted. Most of the toll-free telephone numbers listed in this directory are accessible from every state. Just dial *1 + 800* (or *888*) + *the number.* However, the telephone numbers of some organizations such as poison control centers are accessible only from a single state, portions of a state or a city. For example, the listing for the Poison Center in Omaha, Nebraska, which can be accessed only from Nebraska and Wyoming, is listed:

> The Poison Center
> Omaha, NE
> 800-955-9119 Nebraska and Wyoming

You will also find organizations that have two separate toll-free numbers—one for national use and the other for use in a specific state—as in the following example:

> Shriners Hospital Referral Line
> Tampa, FL
> 800-237-5055
> 800-282-9161 Florida

Some organizations have both a toll-free number and a long-distance (unless, of course, you are calling from within the local area of the number) number listed. This is done in the event that the toll-free number is busy or out of service. These listings appear as follows:

> Neurofibromatosis
> Lanham, MD
> 800-942-6825
> 301-577-8984

Several organizations use their names, initials or another mnemonic device as part of their telephone numbers. In these cases, we have listed both the mnemonic device and the numeric translation to make it easier to dial, as in the following example:

> American International Hospital Cancer Program
> Zion, IL
> 800-FOR-HELP (800-367-4357)

Callers who require services for the hearing- or speech-impaired will find numbers identified by TDD (for use with telecommunications devices) and TTY (for use with teletype devices), as in the following example:

AIDS Hotline
Research Triangle Park, NC
800-243-7889 TDD

The final type of toll-free number found in this directory is the Spanish language line. Some organizations have a dedicated Spanish line, while others offer Spanish on a separate extension, as in the following example:

AIDS Hotline
Research Triangle Park, NC
800-344-7432 Spanish

Hours of operation are listed in local time zones, either eastern, central, mountain or Pacific. There are no references to daylight savings time. Also, many of these organizations are staffed by volunteers who answer the telephone from their homes. Therefore, unless otherwise specified, please be considerate by calling during regular business hours, generally 9:00 A.M. to 5:00 P.M. If you're unsure of the time zone, check the state location on a time zone map, which may be found in your local telephone directory.

With the tremendous growth of on-line services and in-home computers, we've added the e-mail addresses of many organizations. However, be aware that in some cases you may be charged for access to these on-line services, thereby defeating the purpose of toll-free dialing.

Every toll-free number listed in this directory was verified just prior to publication and found to be in operation. However, should you encounter a problem dialing any of the *800* or *888* numbers, we suggest that you call the toll-free directory assistance operator at 800-555-1212.

A brief explanation that describes the type of service or information provided by the organization follows each listing. This will help you to determine whether the organization does indeed provide the kind of information you desire.

The People's Medical Society makes no claims or

guarantees for the organizations listed in this directory. *Dial 800 for Health* is not an endorsement or recommendation of these organizations by the People's Medical Society. We cannot be responsible for the services offered or the content of the information provided. As always, we encourage you to exercise your own good judgment when contacting any of these groups.

ADOPTION

AASK America
657 Mission St., Suite 601
San Francisco, CA 94105
800-232-2751
> *Provides information on how to adopt children with special needs such as those with mental and physical disabilities.*

Child Reach
155 Plan Way
Warwick, RI 02886
800-556-7918
8:45 A.M. to 8:45 P.M. (eastern time), Monday to Friday
> *Provides information on how to become a sponsor to a child living in the Third World.*

Concerned United Birthparents
2000 Walker St.
Des Moines, IA 50317
800-822-2777
515-263-9558 Iowa
24 hours a day, seven days a week
> *Provides information on support groups designed for birth parents who gave up their children for adoption and are now seeking to come to terms with their decision. Also makes referrals to support groups in the caller's area.*

Edna Gladney Center
2300 Hemphill St.
Ft. Worth, TX 76110
800-433-2922
800-772-2740 Texas
8:30 A.M. to 5:00 P.M. (central time), Monday to Saturday
> *Provides counseling and shelter to single pregnant women who want to place their children for adoption. Information packet available upon request.*

International Children's Care
2711 N.E. 134th St.
Vancouver, WA 98686
800-422-7729
> *Provides information to couples or individuals who are interested in international adoptions. Counsels prospective parents on the adoption and immigration laws of the foreign country.*

National Adoption Center
1500 Walnut St.
Philadelphia, PA 19102
800-862-3678
215-925-0200 Philadelphia
9:00 A.M. to 5:00 P.M. (eastern time), Monday to Friday
> *Provides adoption information concerning hard-to-place children and children with special needs.*

Pregnancy Counseling Services
Liberty Godparent Home
Fort Early Building
11 Oakridge Blvd., Suite 201
Lynchburg, VA 24501
800-542-4453
804-384-3043 Virginia
24 hours a day, seven days a week
> *Provides information on residential programs for unwed mothers. Offers counseling and adoption services. Also makes referrals to support groups in the caller's area.*

AEROBIC EXERCISE

Aerobic and Fitness Association of America
15250 Ventura Blvd., Suite 310
Sherman Oaks, CA 91403
800-446-2322
800-445-5950
800-343-2584 California
800-225-2322 Canada and Mexico
8:30 A.M. to 5:00 P.M. (Pacific time), Monday to Friday
> *Provides basic information on aerobic exercise, certified instructors and prevention and treatment of aerobics-related injuries.*

National Dance-Exercise Instructors Training Association
1503 S. Washington Ave., Suite 208
Minneapolis, MN 55454
800-237-6242
612-340-1306 Minnesota
> *Provides information on aerobics instructors and seminars nationwide.*

AIDS
(Acquired Immune Deficiency Syndrome)

AIDS Clinical Trials Information Service
P.O. Box 6421
Rockville, MD 20849–6421
800-874-2572
800-243-7012 TTY
9:00 A.M. to 7:00 P.M. (eastern time), Monday to Friday
e-mail: Actis@cdcnac.aspensys.com
> *Provides information on the status of federally and privately sponsored experimental drug trials for human immunodeficiency virus (HIV) and AIDS. Information packet available upon request.*

AIDS Hotline
c/o American Social Health Association
P.O. Box 13827
Research Triangle Park, NC 27709
800-342-2437
800-243-7889 TDD
24 hours a day, seven days a week
800-344-7432 Spanish
8:00 A.M. to 2:00 A.M. (eastern time), seven days a week
> *Provides information on human immunodeficiency virus (HIV) and AIDS transmission and prevention. Answers specific questions concerning HIV and AIDS. Also makes referrals for testing and counseling. Information packet available upon request.*

American Academy of Pediatrics
Pediatric AIDS Coalition
601 13th St., NW, Suite 400N
Washington, DC 20005
800-336-5475
202-662-7460 District of Columbia
9:00 A.M. to 5:00 P.M. (eastern time), Monday to Friday
> *Provides information on AIDS education programs for adults and children in churches, schools and other community organizations.*

Haitian AIDS Hotline
8037 N.E. Second Ave.
Miami, FL 33138
800-722-7432
8:30 A.M. to 5:00 P.M. (eastern time), Monday to Friday
> *Provides human immunodeficiency virus (HIV) and AIDS information specifically tailored to the Haitian population.*

Multicultural Training Resource Center
1540 Market St., Suite 320
San Francisco, CA 94102
800-545-6642 California
> *Provides human immunodeficiency virus (HIV) and AIDS information specifically targeted to diverse cultural groups.*

Names Project
2362 Market St.
P.O. Box 14573
San Francisco, CA 94114
800-872-6263 California
415-863-5511
9:00 A.M. to 6:00 P.M. (Pacific time), Monday to Friday
> *Provides information on how to add names to the AIDS Memorial Quilt, which commemorates those men, women and children who have lost their lives to AIDS.*

National AIDS Information Clearinghouse
P.O. Box 6003
Rockville, MD 20849–6003
800-458-5231
9:00 A.M. to 7:00 P.M. (eastern time), Monday to Friday
> *Provides recorded messages in English and Spanish with information on organizational and educational materials, clinical drug trials and how to order publications.*

National Native American AIDS Prevention Center
3515 Grand Ave., Suite 100
Oakland, CA 94610
800-283-2437
8:30 A.M. to 5:00 P.M. (Pacific time), Monday to Friday
510-444-2051 Oakland
> *Provides referrals to Native Americans regarding counseling and testing centers. Information packet available upon request.*

People With AIDS Coalition
31 W. 26th St.
New York, NY 10010
800-828-3280
212-532-0290
10:00 A.M. to 6:00 P.M. (eastern time), Monday to Friday
1:00 P.M. to 5:00 P.M. (eastern time), Saturday and Sunday
> *Provides information and referral services to callers. Also provides publications in both English and Spanish.*

Project Inform
220 Market St.
San Francisco, CA 94103
800-822-7422
800-334-7422 California
10:00 A.M. to 4:00 P.M. (Pacific time), Monday to Friday
10:00 A.M. to 1:00 P.M. (Pacific time), Saturday
Answering machine at all other times
> *Provides current information on treatment options for persons with human immunodefiency virus (HIV) and AIDS, as well as information on organizations that provide the treatments. Also operates an outreach and advocacy program.*

Teens Teaching AIDS Prevention
3030 Walnut St.
Kansas City, MO 64108
800-234-8336
816-561-8784 Kansas City
4:00 P.M. to 8:00 P.M. (central time), Monday to Friday
Answering machine at all other times
> *Provides information and counseling on human immunodeficiency virus (HIV) and AIDS from a teen's perspective. Makes referrals to AIDS organizations and other resources. Some literature available at a nominal charge.*

ALLERGIES AND ASTHMA

Allergy and Asthma Network/Mothers of Asthmatics
3554 Chain Bridge Rd., Suite 200
Fairfax, VA 22030
800-878-4403
9:00 A.M. to 5:00 P.M. (eastern time), Monday to Friday
> *Provides patient education and information on asthma and allergy. Sells publications and videos. Individual membership ($25) includes subscription to the* MA Report, *a monthly newsletter.*

Allergy Information Referral Line
American Academy of Allergy and Immunology
611 E. Wells St.
Milwaukee, WI 53202
800-822-2762
414-272-6071 Wisconsin
8:00 A.M. to 5:00 P.M. (central time), Monday to Friday
> *Provides information on the diagnosis and treatment of allergies and asthma. Also makes referrals to allergy specialists.*

American College of Allergy and Immunology
800 W. Northwest Hwy., Suite 1080
Palatine, IL 60067
800-842-7777
24 hours a day, Monday to Friday
> *Provides information on various allergies and the treatment options available.*

Asthma and Allergy Foundation of America
1125 15th St., NW, Suite 502
Washington, DC 20005
800-727-8462
202-466-7643 District of Columbia
> *Provides U.S. maps showing zones where plants are likely to cause allergy problems. Also provides educational materials on asthma and allergies.*

The Food Allergy Network
10400 Eaton Pl., Suite 107
Fairfax, VA 22030–2208
800-929-4040
9:00 A.M. to 5:00 P.M. (eastern time), Monday to Friday
> *Provides information on, and works to increase public awareness of, food allergies. Individual membership ($24) includes a subscription to the bimonthly newsletter* Food Allergy News *and consumer alerts.*

National Jewish Asthma Center
1400 Jackson St.
Denver, CO 80206
800-222-5864
303-398-1477 Denver
8:00 A.M. to 5:00 P.M. (mountain time), Monday to Friday
> *Answers questions about asthma, emphysema, chronic bronchitis and other respiratory diseases. Also makes referrals to doctors in the caller's area. Information packet available upon request.*

ALZHEIMER'S DISEASE

Alzheimer's Association
919 N. Michigan Ave., Suite 1000
Chicago, IL 60611
800-272-3900
8:30 A.M. to 5:00 P.M. (central time), Monday to Friday
Answering machine at all other times
e-mail: Info@alz.org
> *Provides information on Alzheimer's disease and related disorders. Also makes referrals to chapters in the caller's area.*

Alzheimer's Disease Education and Referral Center
National Institute on Aging
Public Information Office
Building 31, Room 5C27
Bethesda, MD 20892
800-438-4380
8:30 A.M. to 5:00 P.M. (eastern time), Monday to Friday
Answering machine at all other times

Provides information on Alzheimer's disease to the public. Also provides information for health professionals. Information packet available upon request.

American Health Assistance Foundation
15825 Shady Grove Rd., Suite 140
Rockville, MD 20850
800-437-2423
301-948-3244 Maryland
9:00 A.M. to 5:00 P.M. (eastern time), Monday to Friday

Provides public education materials on Alzheimer's relief programs and provides funding for such programs. Also provides financial assistance to families in need of relief services.

National Family Caregivers Association
9621 Bexhill Dr.
Kensington, MD 20895–3104
800-896-3650
301-942-6430
9:00 A.M. to 5:00 P.M. (eastern time), Monday to Friday

Provides information and offers support and counseling to individuals who find themselves faced with the responsibility of providing care to a family member.

AMYOTROPHIC LATERAL SCLEROSIS
(ALS; "Lou Gehrig's Disease")

ALS Association
21021 Ventura Blvd., Suite 321
Woodland Hills, CA 91364
800-782-4747
818-340-7500 San Fernando Valley
8:00 A.M. to 5:00 P.M. (Pacific time), Monday to Friday

Provides education, information and referral services to ALS patients and their families. Also makes referrals to chapters in the caller's area.

ANEMIA

Aplastic Anemia Foundation of America
P.O. Box 22689
Baltimore, MD 21203
800-747-2820
410-955-2803 Maryland
9:00 A.M. to 5:00 P.M. (eastern time), Monday to Friday
Provides information and counseling to people with aplastic anemia.

National Association for Sickle Cell Disease
3345 Wilshire Blvd., Suite 1106
Los Angeles, CA 90010–1880
800-421-8453
213-736-5455 Los Angeles
8:30 A.M. to 5:00 P.M. (Pacific time), Monday to Friday
Provides materials, trains counselors and offers programs to medical professionals and the public. Also supports research, conducts public education campaigns and provides diagnostic screening.

ARTHRITIS

Arthritis Consulting Services
4620 N. State Road 7, Suite 206
Ft. Lauderdale, FL 33319
800-327-3027
8:30 A.M. to 4:00 P.M. (eastern time), Monday to Friday
Provides information on holistic approaches to treating arthritis.

Arthritis Foundation Information Line
P.O. Box 19000
Atlanta, GA 30326
800-283-7800
404-872-7100 Georgia
9:00 A.M. to 7:00 P.M. (eastern time), Monday to Friday
Provides physician referrals and information concerning chapters in the caller's area. Information packet available upon request.

Spondylitis Association of America
P.O. Box 5872
Sherman Oaks, CA 92413
800-777-8189
818-981-1616
8:00 A.M. to 5:00 P.M. (Pacific time), Monday to Friday
Answering machine at all other times
e-mail: info@spondylitis.org
> *Provides information on the diagnosis and treatment of the condition.*
> *Also makes referrals to support groups in the caller's area. Information*
> *packet available upon request.*

BEHÇET'S SYNDROME

American Behçet's Association
P.O. Box 27494
Tempe, AZ 85285–7494
800-723-4238
10:00 A.M. to 8:00 P.M. (eastern time), Monday to Friday
e-mail: NYYY49C@Prodigy.com
> *Provides information on this condition to patients and their families.*
> *Also provides mutual support and meets on Prodigy (an on-line*
> *computer service).*

BIRTH-RELATED DISORDERS

American Cleft Palate Educational Foundation
1218 Grandview Ave.
Pittsburgh, PA 15211
800-24-CLEFT (800-242-5338)
800-232-5338 Pennsylvania
7:30 A.M. to 4:30 P.M. (eastern time), Monday to Friday
Answering machine at all other times
> *Provides parents with information on feeding techniques and proper*
> *dental care for children with cleft palates. Also makes referrals to*
> *support groups in the caller's area. Information packet available*
> *upon request.*

Anencephaly Research and Help Line
128 W. Woodstock Circle
Spring, TX 77381
888-206-7526
24 hours a day, seven days a week
> *Provides information and support services to parents with children*
> *who were born anencephalic.*

Association of Birth Defect Children
827 Irma St.
Orlando, FL 32803
800-313-2232
407-245-7035
24 hours a day, seven days a week

> *Provides support services to parents of children with birth defects or developmental disabilities. Maintains birth defects registry that tracks birth defects that may be related to chemical, radiation or other environmental factors. Also operates a referral service that links parents in a support network.*

Autism Society of America
7910 Woodmont Ave., Suite 650
Bethesda, MD 20814
800-328-8476
301-657-0881
9:00 A.M. to 5:00 P.M. (eastern time), Monday to Friday

> *Provides information on the diagnosis and treatment of autism. Promotes public awareness and understanding of adults and children with autism.*

Batten's Disease Support and Research Association
2600 Parsons Ave.
Columbus, OH 43207
800-448-4570
614-445-4161
24 hours a day, seven days a week

> *Provides information and support to families of children afflicted with Batten's disease. Also makes referrals to support groups in the caller's area.*

Beckwith-Wiedemann Syndrome Support Network
3206 Braeburn Circle
Ann Arbor, MI 48108
800-837-2976
313-973-0263
9:00 A.M. to 5:00 P.M. (eastern time), Monday to Friday
Answering machine at all other times

> *Provides information and assistance to families of children with Beckwith-Wiedemann syndrome. Also promotes research into the causes, early diagnosis and treatment of the condition.*

Cornelia de Lange Syndrome (CdLS) Foundation
60 Dyer Ave.
Collinsville, CT 06022
800-223-8355
800-753-2357 Canada
9:00 A.M. to 4:30 P.M. (eastern time), Monday to Friday
Answering machine at all other times
> *Provides general information on the birth defects caused by CdLS.
> Also operates a support system for parents and makes referrals to
> chapters in the caller's area. Information packet available upon request.*

Cystic Fibrosis Foundation
6931 Arlington Rd.
Bethesda, MD 20814
800-344-4823
301-951-4422
8:30 A.M. to 5:30 P.M. (eastern time), Monday to Friday
> *Provides information on cystic fibrosis. Also makes referrals to hospital
> treatment centers and support groups in the caller's area. Information
> packet available upon request.*

Cystinosis Foundation
1212 Broadway
Oakland, CA 94612
800-392-8458
510-235-1052
> *Provides information on the genetic disorder cystinosis and helps to
> raise funds for research. Also provides support to parents of children
> with this condition.*

Fragile X Syndrome
1441 York St., #215
Denver, CO 80206
800-688-8765
303-333-6155
9:00 A.M. to 5:00 P.M. (mountain time), Monday to Friday
Answering machine at all other times
> *Provides information on the detection and treatment of the hereditary
> condition fragile X syndrome. Also provides information on support
> networks and makes referrals in the caller's area.*

International Rett Syndrome Association
9121 Piscataway Rd., #2B
Clinton, MD 20735–2561
800-818-7388
301-856-3334
9:00 A.M. to 5:00 P.M. (eastern time), Monday to Friday
e-mail: irsa@paltech.com
> *Provides information and counseling to parents with children afflicted
> with Rett syndrome. Also promotes and supports research efforts.*

National Down Syndrome Congress
1800 Dempster St.
Park Ridge, IL 60068
800-232-6372
9:00 A.M. to 5:00 P.M. (central time), Monday to Friday
Provides information and referrals on Down syndrome. Publishes a newsletter and sponsors an annual convention.

National Down Syndrome Society
666 Broadway
New York, NY 10012
800-221-4602
9:00 A.M. to 5:00 P.M. (eastern time), Monday to Friday
Answering machine at all other times
Makes referrals to support groups in the caller's area. Publications available for a small fee. Information packet available upon request.

National Gaucher Disease Foundation
11140 Rockville Pike, #350
Rockville, MD 20852–3106
800-925-8885
9:00 A.M. to 5:00 P.M. (eastern time), Monday to Friday
Answering machine at all other times
Provides information and assistance to families with children suffering from Gaucher disease. Also makes referrals to treatment centers and support groups in the caller's area.

Prader-Willi Syndrome Association
2510 S. Brentwood Blvd., #220
St. Louis, MO 63144
800-926-4797
314-962-7644
8:00 A.M. to 4:00 P.M. (central time), Monday to Friday
Answering machine at all other times
e-mail: pwsausa@aol.com
Provides information and support service to parents of children with Prader-Willi syndrome. Information packet available upon request.

Spina Bifida Association of America
4590 MacArthur Blvd., NW, Suite 250
Washington, DC 20007
800-621-3141
301-770-7222 Maryland
9:00 A.M. to 5:00 P.M. (eastern time), Monday to Friday
Answering machine at all other times
Provides information on the birth defect spina bifida. Also makes referrals to chapters in the caller's area.

Sturge-Weber Foundation
P.O. Box 418
Mt. Freedom, NJ 07970
800-627-5482
8:30 A.M. to 2:30 P.M. (eastern time), Monday to Thursday
Answering machine at all other times
> *Provides information on Sturge-Weber syndrome. Operates a mutual support network for families affected by this condition. Also makes referrals in the caller's area. Information packet available upon request.*

Tay-Sachs Foundation
1303 Paper Mill Rd.
Erdenheim, PA 19038
800-672-2022
9:00 A.M. to 5:00 P.M. (eastern time), Monday to Friday
e-mail: 72624.3502E@Compuserve.com
> *Provides information on Tay-Sachs disease as well as advocacy and support for families with children affected by this genetic condition. Also makes referrals to support groups in the caller's area.*

Turner's Syndrome Society
814 Glencarin Ave.
Toronto, Ontario
Canada M6B 2A3
800-465-6744
416-781-2086
24 hours a day, seven days a week
> *Provides information and support to families affected by Turner's syndrome. Also makes referrals to Canadian and U.S. support groups in the caller's area.*

Turner's Syndrome Society of the United States
1313 S.E. Fifth St., Suite 327
Minneapolis, MN 55414
800-365-9944
612-379-3607
8:30 A.M. to 5:00 P.M. (central time), Monday to Friday
e-mail: Tesch005@tc.umn.edu
> *Provides information on Turner's syndrome. Also works to increase public awareness and support for research into the causes and prevention of this genetic disorder affecting females. Information packet available upon request.*

United Cerebral Palsy Association
1522 K St., NW, Suite 1112
Washington, DC 20005
800-872-5827
202-842-1266
9:00 A.M. to 5:00 P.M. (eastern time), Monday to Friday
> *Provides information on the diagnosis and treatment of cerebral palsy. Works to establish local programs that help people with the disease move into mainstream society.*

BLOOD DISORDERS

National Hemophilia Foundation
110 Greene St., Suite 303
New York, NY 10012
800-424-2634
212-431-8541
9:00 A.M. to 5:00 P.M. (eastern time), Monday to Friday
Answering machine at all other times
> *Provides information and referrals to families affected by hemophilia. Also supports research and disseminates information to raise the public awareness about hemophilia.*

National Marrow Donor Program
3433 Broadway St., NE, Suite 400
Minneapolis, MN 55413–1762
800-654-1247 Extension 149 for Spanish
8:00 A.M. to 6:00 P.M. (central time), Monday to Friday
Answering machine at all other times
> *Maintains a registry of bone marrow donors. Also provides information on how interested individuals can become active in the registry program.*

BURN CARE

Phoenix Society
National Organization for Burn Survivors
11 Rust Hill Rd.
Levittown, PA 19056
800-888-2876
215-946-4788
> *Provides information on the self-help services available to burn victims and their families. Helps burn victims deal with their trauma and provides the psychological support they need to return to normal lives and interests. Information packet available upon request.*

Shriners Hospital Referral Line
2900 Rocky Point Dr.
Tampa, FL 33607–1435
800-237-5055
800-282-9161 Florida
8:00 A.M. to 5:00 P.M. (eastern time), Monday to Friday
> *Provides information on burn treatment programs available at*
> *Shriners hospitals.*

CANCER

AMC Cancer Information and Counseling Line
American Medical Center
1600 Pierce St.
Denver, CO 80214
800-525-3777
303-233-6501 Denver
8:30 A.M. to 4:45 P.M. (mountain time), Monday to Friday
> *Provides the latest information on cancer prevention, detection and*
> *treatment methods. Offers counseling. Also makes referrals to support*
> *groups in the caller's area.*

American Association of Oral and Maxillofacial Surgeons
9700 Bryn Mawr Ave.
Rosemont, IL 60018
800-467-5268
8:30 A.M. to 5:00 P.M. (central time), Monday to Friday
Answering machine at all other times
> *Provides information on oral cancer. Also makes referrals to oral*
> *surgeons in the caller's area.*

American Brain Tumor Association
2720 River Rd., Suite 146
Des Plaines, IL 60018
800-886-2282
847-827-9910
e-mail: ABTA@aol.com
> *Provides information on brain tumors and support groups in the*
> *caller's area. Encourages and supports research efforts aimed at*
> *treating brain tumors.*

American Cancer Society
1599 Clifton Rd., NE
Atlanta, GA 30329
800-227-2345
8:30 A.M. to 4:30 P.M. (eastern time), Monday to Friday
Provides general information on the society's programs and services. Makes referrals to chapters in the caller's area. Also answers questions about cancer, including those regarding prevention, diagnosis, treatment and rehabilitation.

American International Hospital Cancer Program
2501 Emmaus Ave.
Zion, IL 60099
800-FOR-HELP (800-367-4357)
708-872-4561
Provides information on cancer treatment programs available at hospitals.

Cancer Care
1180 Avenue of the Americas
New York, NY 10036
800-813-4673 Extension 2 for Spanish
e-mail: info@cancercareinc.org
Provides information and counseling to cancer patients and their families. Also makes referrals to support groups in the caller's area.

Cancer Research Institute
681 Fifth Ave.
New York, NY 10022
800-992-2623
9:00 A.M. to 5:00 P.M. (eastern time), Monday to Friday
Answering machine at all other times
e-mail: info@cancerresearch.org
Provides information on recent developments in the diagnosis, treatment and prevention of cancer.

Candlelighters Childhood Cancer Foundation
7910 Woodmont Ave., Suite 460
Bethesda, MD 20814
800-366-2223
24 hours a day, seven days a week
Provides information and services such as a 24-hour crisis line and transportation to families of childhood cancer patients. Serves as a clearinghouse and liaison between parents and medical professionals. Establishes Ronald McDonald houses, where family members of patients may stay while the patient undergoes treatment.

CHEMOcare

231 North Ave., W
Westfield, NJ 07090
800-55-CHEMO (800-552-4366)
908-233-1103 New Jersey
9:00 A.M. to 5:30 P.M. (eastern time), Monday to Friday
Answering machine at all other times
e-mail: chemocare@aol.com

> *Provides information and support to cancer patients who are currently undergoing chemotherapy or radiation therapy. Operates a one-on-one emotional support network for these patients.*

Comprehensive Cancer Center

University of Alabama at Birmingham
University Station
Birmingham, AL 35294
800-UAB-0933 (800-822-0933)
205-934-5077

> *Provides information on cancer treatment programs available at the university center.*

International Cancer Alliance

4853 Cordell Ave., Suite 11
Bethesda, MD 20814
800-422-7361
9:00 A.M. to 5:00 P.M. (eastern time), Monday to Friday
Answering machine at all other times

> *Provides free information on various types of cancers, including diagnostic tests, staging and treatments. Also publishes quarterly reports on progress against cancer.*

International Myeloma Foundation

2120 Stanley Hills Dr.
Los Angeles, CA 90046
800-452-2873
213-654-3023
8:00 A.M. to 5:00 P.M. (Pacific time), Monday to Friday
Answering machine at all other times
e-mail: TheIMF@aol.com

> *Provides information to patients and professionals on the diagnosis and treatment of myeloma. Supports research and sponsors conferences. Also publishes a quarterly newsletter.*

Leukemia Society of America
600 Third Ave.
New York, NY 10016
800-955-4572
212-573-8484
24 hours a day, seven days a week
> *Provides information on the latest research into the causes and treatment of leukemia and related cancers. Also sponsors national programs on patient and professional education.*

Make Today Count
Mid-American Cancer Center
1235 E. Cherokee St.
Springfield, MO 65804–2263
800-432-2273
417-885-2000
9:00 A.M. to 4:30 P.M. (central time), Monday to Friday
Answering machine at all other times
> *Provides information on this mutual support organization, that helps people affected by life-threatening illnesses to lead full and complete lives. Encourages mutual support and self-help.*

Mathews Foundation for Prostate Cancer Research
817 Commons Dr.
Sacramento, CA 95825
800-234-6284
916-567-1400
e-mail: mathews@sna.com
> *Provides information on the symptoms, diagnosis and treatment of prostate cancer. Also responds to individual questions concerning the effects of the disease.*

National Alliance of Breast Cancer Organizations
9 E. 37th St., 10th Floor
New York, NY 10016
800-719-9154
24 hours a day, seven days a week
e-mail: NABCOinfo@aol.com
> *Provides information on breast cancer. Also serves as an advocate for legislation and regulatory concerns of breast cancer patients and their families.*

National Brain Tumor Foundation
785 Market St., Suite 1600
San Francisco, CA 94103
800-934-2873
415-284-0208
9:00 A.M. to 5:00 P.M. (Pacific time), Monday to Friday
Answering machine at all other times
> *Provides information on the latest research into discovering an effective treatment for brain tumors. Also makes referrals to support groups in the caller's area.*

National Cancer Institute
Cancer Information Service
9000 Rockville Pike, Suite 414
Bethesda, MD 20892
800-422-6237
800-638-6070 Alaska
800-524-1234 Hawaii
9:00 A.M. to 10:00 P.M. (eastern time), Monday to Friday
> *Provides information on various types of cancers and the latest treatments available for those cancers. Information packets in both English and Spanish available upon request.*

Nutrition Hotline
American Institute for Cancer Research
1759 R St., NW
Washington, DC 20009
800-843-8114
202-328-7744 District of Columbia
9:00 A.M. to 9:00 P.M. (eastern time), Monday to Thursday
9:00 A.M. to 5:00 P.M. (eastern time), Friday
Answering machine at all other times
> *Provides information on the role of diet and nutrition in cancer prevention and how nutrition may be used to assist a cancer treatment program. Also responds to specific requests for information.*

The Skin Cancer Foundation
P.O. Box 561
New York, NY 10156
800-754-6490
212-725-5176
24 hours a day, seven days a week
> *Provides educational materials on skin cancer. Also conducts seminars to help reduce the incidence of skin cancer.*

Susan G. Komen Breast Cancer Foundation
5005 LBJ Freeway, Suite 370
Dallas, TX 75244
800-462-9273
24 hours a day, seven days a week

> *Provides information on general breast health, including information on breast cancer. Supports events that raise money to research the causes of breast cancer. Also makes referrals to chapters in the caller's area.*

Y-ME
National Breast Cancer Organization
212 W. Van Buren, 5th Floor
Chicago, IL 60607
800-221-2141
24 hours a day, seven days a week
800-986-9505 Spanish
9:00 A.M. to 5:00 P.M. (central time), Monday to Friday

> *Provides information and support to women undergoing treatment for breast cancer. Also provides information on prostheses after breast surgery.*

CHILDREN'S SERVICES

American Academy of Pediatrics
P.O. Box 927
141 N.W. Point Blvd.
Elk Grove, IL 60007
800-433-9016
800-421-0589 Illinois

> *Provides information on pediatric care and the role of the pediatrician.*

American Association for Protecting Children
Division of American Humane Association
63 Inverness Dr., E
Englewood, CO 80112
800-227-5242
303-792-9900 Colorado
8:30 A.M. to 5:00 P.M. (mountain time), Monday to Friday
Answering machine at all other times

> *Provides services to professionals who work in the child protection field. Also conducts research and program evaluations of child welfare agencies. Information packet available upon request.*

Boystown Hotline
Father Flanagan's Boystown
Boystown, NE 68010
800-448-3000
24 hours a day, seven days a week
*Provides assistance to runaway and homeless children regardless of
race, color or creed.*

Child Find Hotline
P.O. Box 277
New Paltz, NY 12561
800-426-5678
914-255-1848 New York
24 hours a day, seven days a week
*Operates an international locator service for missing and abducted
children. Also maintains a registry of missing children.*

Children's Defense Fund
122 C St., NW, Suite 400
Washington, DC 20001
800-CDF-1200 (800-233-1200)
202-628-8787 District of Columbia
9:00 A.M. to 5:00 P.M. (eastern time), Monday to Friday
*Provides information on the expanding field of children's rights as
recognized by law and is involved in social and educational programs
affecting children. Information packet available upon request.*

Children's Wish Foundation
7840 Roswell Rd., Suite 301
Atlanta, GA 30350
800-323-9474
404-393-9474 Georgia
9:00 A.M. to 5:00 P.M. (eastern time), Monday to Friday
*Provides information on programs that seek to grant a dying child his
or her final wish. Works with organizations and individuals who want
to become Wish Foundation supporters.*

Covenant House
460 W. 41st St.
New York, NY 10036
800-999-9999
24 hours a day, seven days a week
*Provides assistance to runaways and homeless youth. Also provides
temporary shelter until the child's situation at home can be resolved.*

Feingold Association of the United States
P.O. Box 6550
Alexandria, VA 22306
800-321-3287
24 hours a day, seven days a week

> *Provides information on the Feingold Program, which uses diet to treat children with learning and behavioral problems. Also makes referrals to support groups in the caller's area. Information packet available upon request.*

Human Growth Foundation
7777 Leesburg Pike
Falls Church, VA 22043
800-451-6434
703-883-1773
8:30 A.M. to 5:00 P.M. (eastern time), Monday to Friday
Answering machine at all other times

> *Makes referrals to chapters on growth disorders in the caller's area. Information packets available upon request.*

Informed Parents Against VAPP
(vaccine-associated paralytic polio)
P.O. Box 53212
Washington, DC 20009
888-363-8277

> *Provides information to families who have been affected by vaccine-associated paralytic polio as a result of immunization. Helps parents network and exchange information.*

"Just Say No" Kids Club International
2101 Webster St., Suite 1300
Oakland, CA 94612
800-258-2766
510-939-6666

> *Provides information on drug prevention programs for children and on how to start a "Just Say No" chapter.*

Kevin Collins Foundation for Missing Children
P.O. Box 590473
San Francisco, CA 94159
800-272-0012

> *Provides counseling and education to the families of missing or abducted children and helps them through the ordeal.*

Kidsrights
10100 Park Cedar Dr.
Charlotte, NC 28210
800-892-5437
8:30 A.M. to 5:00 P.M. (eastern time), Monday to Friday
Provides information to parents and other interested individuals on how to establish programs that work to combat teen suicide.

Little People of America
7238 Piedmont Dr.
Dallas, TX 75227–9324
800-24-DWARF (800-243-9273)
214-388-9576
9:00 A.M. to 5:00 P.M. (central time), Monday to Friday
Provides information and support to children, teens and young adults who are vertically challenged. Promotes fellowship and an exchange of ideas on how to cope with physical and emotional problems.

Missing Children Awareness Foundation
13094 95th St., N
Largo, FL 34643
800-741-7233
Provides assistance and referrals to parents of missing children.

Missing Children Help Center
410 Ware Blvd., Suite 400
Tampa, FL 33619
800-872-5437
Provides assistance to parents of missing children by publicizing the children's photographs in newspapers, brochures and flyers.

National Association for the Education of Young Children
1834 Connecticut Ave., NW
Washington, DC 20009
800-424-2460
9:00 A.M. to 5:00 P.M. (eastern time), Monday to Friday
Provides information and referrals to accredited child-care programs.

National Child Watch Campaign
P.O. Box 1368
Jackson, MI 49204
800-222-1464
Provides information on child safety and how to establish a child-watch program to protect children from being kidnapped. Also provides counseling and support services to parents whose children have been kidnapped or are missing.

National Hotline for Missing and Exploited Children
2101 Wilson Blvd., Suite 550
Arlington, VA 22201
800-843-5678
7:30 A.M. to 11:00 P.M. (eastern time), Monday to Friday
10:00 A.M. to 6:00 P.M. (eastern time), Saturday

Operates a hotline for reporting sightings of missing children and children exploited by crime, prostitution and pornography. Provides technical assistance to legal authorities in the hunt for missing or kidnapped children.

National Information Clearinghouse for Infants
With Disabilities and Life-Threatening Conditions
University of South Carolina
Benson Building, 1st Floor
Columbia, SC 29208
800-922-9234 Voice and TDD
800-922-1107 Voice and TDD South Carolina
9:00 A.M. to 5:00 P.M. (eastern time), Monday to Friday
Answering machine at all other times

Provides information to families with children who have rare or life-threatening conditions. Also offers referrals to professional and community services in the caller's area. Offers special services to Vietnam veterans and their families.

National Resource Center on Child Sexual Abuse
107 Lincoln St.
Huntsville, AL 35801
800-543-7006

Provides resources to agencies dealing with children who have been sexually abused. Also provides bibliographies and articles on the sexual abuse of children.

National Runaway Hotline
Office of the Governor
P.O. Box 12428
Austin, TX 78711
800-231-6946
800-392-3352 Texas

Provides assistance to runaway children by making referrals to shelters and other agencies. Also delivers messages to the families of runaway children.

National Runaway Switchboard
3080 N. Lincoln Ave.
Chicago, IL 60657
800-621-4000
24 hours a day, seven days a week

Provides counseling and referrals to runaway youths 18 years of age and younger.

Operation Lookout
National Center for Missing Youth
P.O. Box 231
Mount Lake Terrace, WA 98043
800-782-7335
> *Provides assistance in locating missing children.*

Parent Help Line
Nashua Brookside Hospital
11 Northwest Blvd.
Nashua, NH 03063
800-543-6381
> *Provides referrals to organizations that can aid parents in obtaining*
> *treatment and counseling for troubled children.*

Shriners Hospital Referral Line
2900 Rocky Point Dr.
Tampa, FL 33607–1435
800-237-5055
800-282-9161 Florida
8:00 A.M. to 5:00 P.M. (eastern time), Monday to Friday
> *Provides information on children's services available at*
> *Shriners hospitals.*

Teen Crisis Hotline
498 S. Spring St.
Crestview, FL 32536
800-262-8336 Florida
> *Provides information and referrals to teenagers facing crises*
> *in their lives.*

Toughlove International
P.O. Box 1069
Doylestown, PA 18901
800-333-1069
215-348-7090 Pennsylvania
> *Serves as a support group for parents of teenage children with*
> *behavioral problems. Makes referrals in both the United States*
> *and Canada.*

Vanished Children's Alliance
1407 Parkmoor Ave., Suite 200
San Jose, CA 95126
800-826-4743
408-971-4822
24 hours a day, seven days a week
> *Provides information on missing and recovered children.*

Youth Crisis Hotline
10225 Ulmerton Rd., Suite 4-A
Largo, FL 34641
800-442-4673
> *Provides information on child abuse. Also serves as an advocacy group for abused children.*

CHRONIC FATIGUE SYNDROME

Chronic Fatigue Immune Dysfunction Syndrome (CFIDS) Association
P.O. Box 220398
Charlotte, NC 28222–0398
800-442-3437
24 hours a day, seven days a week
> *Provides information and educational materials on the effects of chronic fatigue syndrome. Also supports and funds research.*

DENTAL CARE

American Academy of Cosmetic Dentistry
2711 Marshall Ct.
Madison, WI 53705
800-543-9220
> *Provides information on cosmetic dentistry. Also makes referrals to practitioners in the caller's area.*

Environmental Dental Association
9974 Scripps Ranch Blvd., Suite 36
San Diego, CA 92131
800-388-8124
> *Provides information on alternatives to mercury fillings and how to locate dentists who do not use mercury fillings.*

DIABETES MELLITUS

American Diabetes Association
1660 Duke St.
Alexandria, VA 22314
800-232-3472
703-549-1500
8:30 A.M. to 5:00 P.M. (eastern time), Monday to Friday
> *Provides general information on the diagnosis and treatment of diabetes. Information packet available upon request.*

Juvenile Diabetes Foundation
120 Wall St., 19th Floor
New York, NY 10005
800-223-1138
212-889-7575
9:00 A.M. to 5:00 P.M. (eastern time), Monday to Friday
e-mail: Info@jufcure.com
> *Provides information on the latest research into the causes and prevention of juvenile diabetes. Also provides grants to support ongoing research.*

DIGESTIVE DISEASES

Crohn's and Colitis Foundation
444 Park Ave., S
New York, NY 10018
800-343-3637
9:00 A.M. to 5:00 P.M. (eastern time), Monday to Friday
> *Provides information on digestive diseases and their diagnosis and treatment. Also makes referrals to support groups and chapters in the caller's area. Information packet available upon request.*

DISABLED PERSONS' SERVICES

American Paralysis Association
500 Morris Ave.
Springfield, NJ 07081
800-225-0292
800-526-3456 New Jersey
8:30 A.M. to 5:00 P.M. (eastern time), Monday to Friday
> *Provides information on the treatment of spinal cord injuries. Also makes referrals to support groups in the caller's area. Information packet available upon request.*

Architectural and Transportation Barriers Compliance Board
1111 18th St., NW, Suite 501
Washington, DC 20036
800-USA-ABLE (800-872-2253) Voice and TDD
9:00 A.M. to 5:00 P.M. (eastern time), Monday to Friday
> *Provides information to businesses and other organizations on how to comply with the public accommodations guidelines of the Americans With Disabilities Act as required by Title III.*

AT&T National Special Needs Center
2001 Route 46, Suite 310
Parsippany, NJ 07054
800-872-3883
800-833-3232 TDD
8:30 A.M. to 6:30 P.M. (eastern time), Monday to Friday

Provides information on purchasing or renting special equipment and services available to people with hearing, speech, vision or motion impairment.

Devereux Foundation
19 S. Waterloo Rd.
Devon, PA 19333
800-345-1292 Extension 3109
8:45 A.M. to 9:00 P.M. (eastern time), Monday to Friday

Provides information on treatment programs for children, adolescents and adults with psychiatric, emotional, neurological and developmental disabilities. Information packet available upon request.

Equal Employment Opportunity Commission
1801 L St., NW
Washington, DC 20507
800-669-EEOC (800-669-3362)
800-800-3302 TDD
9:00 A.M. to 5:00 P.M. (eastern time), Monday to Friday

Provides information to businesses and other organizations on how to comply with the equal employment opportunity requirements of the Americans With Disabilities Act as required by Title I.

IBM National Support Center for People With Disabilities
P.O. Box 2150
Atlanta, GA 30301
800-426-2133

Provides information on how computers can be used to assist persons with disabilities.

Institute of Logopedics
2400 Jardine Dr.
Wichita, KS 67219
800-835-1043
800-937-4644 Canada
8:00 A.M. to 5:00 P.M. (central time), Monday to Friday

Provides information on residential programs for children with multiple disabilities.

Job Accommodation Network
809 Allen Hall
P.O. Box 6123
West Virginia University
Morgantown, WV 26506–6123
800-526-7234
800-526-4698 West Virginia
> *Provides information to employers and the public on how to accommodate the needs of persons with disabilities in the workplace.*

National Association of Rehabilitation Facilities
P.O. Box 17675
Washington, DC 20041
800-368-3513
8:30 A.M. to 5:30 P.M. (eastern time), Monday to Friday
Answering machine at all other times
> *Provides the names and locations of rehabilitation facilities. Also makes referrals to support groups in the caller's area.*

National Center for Youth With Disabilities
University of Minnesota, Box 721
420 Delaware St., NE
Minneapolis, MN 55455
800-333-6293
612-624-3939 TDD
7:45 A.M. to 4:30 P.M. (central time), Monday to Friday
> *Provides information to assist parents, educators, caregivers, advocates and others in helping children and youth with disabilities to become fully participating members of society.*

National Clearinghouse on Postsecondary Education for Individuals With Disabilities
1 DuPont Circle, Suite 800
Washington, DC 20036–1193
800-544-3284
202-939-9320 District of Columbia
> *Provides information for individuals with disabilities on job opportunities following graduation from high school.*

National Easter Seal Society
230 W. Monroe St., Suite 1800
Chicago, IL 60606–4802
800-221-6827
8:30 A.M. to 5:00 P.M. (central time), Monday to Friday
> *Provides information on therapy, counseling and educational programs for persons with disabilities. Also makes referrals to community-based programs in the caller's area.*

National Information Center for Children and Youth With Disabilities

P.O. Box 1492
Washington, DC 20013
800-695-0285
202-884-8200
9:30 A.M. to 6:30 P.M. (eastern time), Monday to Friday
Answering machine at all other times
e-mail: NICHCY@aed.org

Provides information on programs for children and youth with disabilities.

National Rehabilitation Information Center

8455 Colesville Rd., Suite 935
Silver Spring, MD 20910–3319
800-346-2742
8:00 A.M. to 6:00 P.M. (eastern time), Monday to Friday

Provides information on resources and products for persons with disabilities. Also provides information on research databases that may be used by persons with disabilities.

National Tour Association

Handicapped Travel Division
546 E. Main St.
Lexington, KY 40508
800-682-8886

Provides information to travelers who require special accommodations because of disabilities or other limitations. Provides a list of travel operators who book accommodations for individuals with disabilities.

Pathways Awareness Foundation

123 N. Wacker Dr.
Chicago, IL 60606
800-955-2445
9:00 A.M. to 5:00 P.M. (central time), Monday to Friday

Provides information on the detection of disabilities in early childhood.

Tele-Consumer Hotline

1910 K St., NW, Suite 610
Washington, DC 20006
800-332-1124

Assists persons with disabilities in locating communications equipment that can be adapted to their individual needs.

DOMESTIC VIOLENCE/SEXUAL ABUSE

Hit Home Youth Crisis Line
Youth Development International
P.O. Box 178408
San Diego, CA 92177–8408
800-448-4663
619-292-5683
> *Provides counseling and referrals on child abuse, runaways, suicide, molestation and pregnancy.*

National Child Abuse Hotline
ChildHelp USA
P.O. Box 630
Hollywood, CA 90028
800-422-4453
24 hours a day, seven days a week
> *Provides crisis counseling and intervention for any abuse-related situation. Also offers information and referral service that includes national, regional or local organizations, agencies and groups. Information packet available upon request.*

National Council on Child Abuse and Family Violence
1155 Connecticut Ave., NW, Suite 300
Washington, DC 20036
800-222-2000
202-429-6695 District of Columbia
7:30 A.M. to 4:30 P.M. (eastern time), Monday to Friday
> *Provides referrals to community services and support groups in the caller's area. Information packet available upon request.*

National Resource Center on Child Sexual Abuse
107 Lincoln St.
Huntsville, AL 35801
800-543-7006
> *Provides resources to agencies dealing with children who have been sexually abused. Also provides bibliographies and articles on the sexual abuse of children.*

Parents Anonymous/Abusive Parents
520 S. Lafayette Park Pl., Suite 316
Los Angeles, CA 90057
800-421-0353
800-352-0386 California
8:30 A.M. to 5:00 P.M. (Pacific time), Monday to Friday
Answering machine at all other times
> *Provides information on the prevention and treatment of child abuse. Also makes referrals to self-help groups and chapters in the caller's area.*

DRINKING WATER

GEO/Resource Consultant
1555 Wilson Blvd., Suite 500
Arlington, VA 22209
800-426-4791
8:00 A.M. to 5:00 P.M. (eastern time), Monday to Friday
> *Provides information on drinking water standards that must be met by community and municipal water suppliers.*

DYSLEXIA

Orton Dyslexia Society
Chester Building, Suite 382
8600 LaSalle Rd.
Baltimore, MD 21286–2044
800-222-3123
410-296-0232 Baltimore
9:00 A.M. to 5:00 P.M. (eastern time), Monday to Friday
> *Provides information on support networks and resources for people with dyslexia.*

EATING DISORDERS

Camelback Helpline
7575 E. Earl Dr.
Scottsdale, AZ 85251
800-253-1334
24 hours a day, seven days a week
> *Provides information on subjects such as mental health, eating disorders and substance dependency. Also makes referrals to treatment centers in the caller's area. Information packet available upon request.*

FIT-AHL
Food Addiction Hotline
2000 Commerce St.
Melbourne, FL 32904
800-872-0088
8:00 A.M. to 9:00 P.M. (eastern time), Monday to Friday
9:00 A.M. to 6:00 P.M. (eastern time), Saturday and Sunday
> *Provides information on eating disorders. Also makes referrals to services in the caller's area. Information packet available upon request.*

Take Off Pounds Sensibly (TOPS)
P.O. Box 07630
4575 S. Fifth St.
Milwaukee, WI 53207
800-932-8677
24 hours a day, seven days a week
> *Provides information on a sensible approach to weight control by showing individuals how to set realistic goals for weight reduction. Also makes referrals to support groups in the caller's area.*

EMERGENCY MEDICAL COMMUNICATION SYSTEMS

American Medical Alert Corporation
3265 Lawson Blvd.
Oceanside, NY 11572
800-645-3244
> *Provides information on telecommunication devices that are used by people with life-threatening conditions or, in the case of accidents, that are used to summon help in emergency situations.*

Lifeline Systems
1 Arsenal Marketplace
Watertown, MA 02172
800-451-0525
617-923-4141 Alaska, Hawaii and Massachusetts
> *Provides information on communication systems that link elderly persons and persons with disabilities directly to hospitals.*

ENDOMETRIOSIS

Endometriosis Association
8585 N. 76th Pl.
Milwaukee, WI 53223
800-992-3636
800-426-2363 Canada
24 hours a day, seven days a week
> *Provides information on the diagnosis and treatment of endometriosis.*

Endometriosis Treatment Program
St. Charles Medical Center
2500 N.E. Neff Rd.
Bend, OR 97701
800-446-2177 Extension 6904
541-382-8622
9:00 A.M. to 5:00 P.M. (Pacific time), Monday to Friday
> *Provides information on the diagnosis and treatment of endometriosis. Offers support and counseling to callers.*

ENTERAL/PARENTERAL NUTRITION

Oley Foundation
214 HUN Memorial
Albany Medical Center A-23
Albany, NY 12208
800-776-6539
518-262-5079
9:00 A.M. to 5:00 P.M. (eastern time), Monday to Friday
Answering machine at all other times
> *Provides information on this specialized system of nutritional therapy to individuals and their families. Publishes a newsletter. Also makes referrals to support groups in the caller's area.*

EPILEPSY

Epilepsy Foundation of America
4351 Garden City Dr.
Landover, MD 20785
800-332-1000
9:00 A.M. to 6:00 P.M. (eastern time), Monday to Friday
> *Provides information on the diagnosis and treatment of epilepsy. Makes referrals to practitioners in the caller's area. Also operates a discount pharmacy available to members.*

FACIAL DISFIGUREMENT

About Face USA
P.O. Box 737
Warrington, PA 18976
800-225-3223
24 hours a day, seven days a week
> *Provides information and support to people with facial disfigurements. Also makes referrals to support groups in the caller's area.*

Forward Face
317 E. 34th St., 9th Floor
New York, NY 10016
800-393-3223
212-263-6656
9:00 A.M. to 4:00 P.M. (eastern time), Monday to Friday
Answering machine at all other times

Provides information on craniofacial disorders and support services available. Also maintains links with medical practitioners and publishes a newsletter.

HANSON'S DISEASE

American Leprosy Missions
1 American Leprosy Mission Way
Greenville, SC 29601
800-543-3131
8:00 A.M. to 5:00 P.M. (eastern time), Monday to Friday

Provides information on the diagnosis and treatment of Hanson's disease. Also makes referrals to treatment programs. Information packet available upon request.

HEADACHE

American Council for Headache Education
875 Kings Hwy., Suite 200
West Deptford, NJ 08096
800-255-2243
609-384-8760
24 hours a day, seven days a week

Provides information on the latest research into the causes of headache. Also publishes brochures and patient education materials.

National Headache Foundation
428 W. St. James Pl., 2nd Floor
Chicago, IL 60614
800-843-2256
9:00 A.M. to 5:00 P.M. (central time), Monday to Friday

Provides general information on the diagnosis and treatment of headache. Also makes referrals to support groups in the caller's area.

New England Headache Treatment Program
778 Longridge Rd.
Stamford, CT 06902
800-245-0088
203-968-1799 Connecticut
9:00 A.M. to 4:00 P.M. (eastern time), Monday to Friday
Provides general information on headache and treatment programs available at Greenwich Hospital in Greenwich, Connecticut. Information packet available upon request.

HEAD INJURY

National Head Injury Foundation
1776 Massachusetts Ave., NW, Suite 100
Washington, DC 20036
800-444-6443
202-296-6443 District of Columbia
9:00 A.M. to 5:00 P.M. (eastern time), Monday to Friday
Provides information on the treatment of head injuries. Also makes referrals to support groups in the caller's area.

HEALTH INFORMATION

Agency for Health Care Policy and Research (AHCPR)
U.S. Department of Health and Human Services
AHCPR Publications Clearinghouse
P.O. Box 8547
Silver Spring, MD 20907
800-358-9295
888-586-6340 TDD
410-381-3150
9:00 A.M. to 5:00 P.M. (eastern time), Monday to Friday
Provides information on publications available from the AHCPR dealing with health research studies funded by the federal government. Some publications are available free of charge.

American Institute for Preventive Medicine
30445 Northwestern Hwy.
Farmington Hills, MI 48075
800-345-2476
313-539-1800 Michigan
8:30 A.M. to 5:30 P.M. (eastern time), Monday to Friday
Provides information on programs designed for lifestyle improvement such as stress reduction, weight control, smoking cessation and health education. Information packet available upon request.

American Medical Radio News

515 N. State St.
Chicago, IL 60610
800-448-9384

> *Provides a recorded message on a current health topic or feature story in medicine.*

American Osteopathic Association

142 E. Ontario St.
Chicago, IL 60611
800-621-1773
312-280-5800
8:30 A.M. to 4:30 P.M. (central time), Monday to Friday

> *Provides information on osteopathic medicine. Also makes referrals to osteopathic physicians and medical centers in the caller's area.*

American Trauma Society

8903 Presidential Pkwy., Suite 512
Upper Marlboro, MD 20772–2656
800-556-7890
301-420-4189
9:00 A.M. to 5:00 P.M. (eastern time), Monday to Friday

> *Provides information on injury prevention and trauma care. Information packet available upon request.*

California Self-Help Center

UCLA Psychology Department
405 Hilgard Ave.
Los Angeles, CA 90024
800-222-5465 California

> *Provides consumer information on a variety of health topics. Also makes referrals to local, regional and national organizations.*

Center for Self Help

Riverwood Center
P.O. Box 547
Benton Harbor, MI 49022–0547
800-336-0341 Michigan

> *Provides information on self-help resources available in the caller's area.*

Consumer Health Information Resource Institute

3521 Broadway
Kansas City, MO 64111
800-821-6671
816-753-8850
9:00 A.M. to 5:00 P.M. (central time), Monday to Friday

> *Provides referrals to local, regional and national organizations. Also maintains a patient education library. Recommends sources of health information on various conditions, procedures and medications.*

Doctor Referral Service of Mt. Sinai Medical Center
1 Gustave L. Levy Pl.
P.O. Box 1083
New York, NY 10029–6575
800-637-4624
8:30 A.M. to 6:00 P.M. (eastern time), Monday to Friday
> *Provides referrals to physicians located in the New York City area who are affiliated with Mt. Sinai Medical Center.*

Food and Drug Administration
Office of Consumer Affairs
Parklawn Building
5600 Fishers Ln.
Rockville, MD 20857
800-532-4440
9:00 A.M. to 5:00 P.M. (eastern time), Monday to Friday
> *Provides information to consumers on Food and Drug Administration actions relative to food and drug items. Also provides consumer education publications and responds to public inquiries.*

Health Information Network International
4213 Montgomery Dr.
Santa Rosa, CA 95405
800-743-6996
707-539-3966
9:00 A.M. to 5:00 P.M. (Pacific time), Monday to Friday
> *Provides consumers with the latest research and information on natural health substances, medical conditions and treatment alternatives.*

International Chiropractic Association
1110 N. Glebe Rd.
Arlington, VA 22201
800-423-4690
> *Provides information on the practice of "straight" chiropractic, which emphasizes spinal manipulation and does not incorporate adjunctive therapies such as heat, cold, ultrasound or vitamins and minerals.*

Joseph and Rose Kennedy Institute of Ethics
National Reference Center for Bioethics Literature
Georgetown University
Washington, DC 20057
800-633-3849
202-687-3885
> *Provides information to medical professionals and the public on medical bioethics.*

National Health Information Center
U.S. Department of Health and Human Services
Office of Disease Prevention and Health Promotion
P.O. Box 1133
Washington, DC 20013
800-336-4797
301-565-4167 Maryland
9:00 A.M. to 5:00 P.M. (eastern time), Monday to Friday
> *Provides information to consumers and professionals on a variety of health-related topics. Also makes referrals to national organizations in the caller's area. Information packet available upon request.*

National Institute for Occupational Safety and Health
Department of Health and Human Resources
4676 Columbia Pkwy.
Cincinnati, OH 45226
800-356-4674
24 hours a day, seven days a week
> *Provides information on workplace safety and compliance with federal occupational and safety regulations.*

National Library of Medicine
8600 Rockville Pike, 4th Floor
Bethesda, MD 20894
800-638-8480
> *Provides information on the services offered at the National Library of Medicine, including computer access to medical literature and information-retrieval systems.*

New Jersey Self-Help Clearinghouse
Northwest Covenant Medical Center
25 Pocono Rd.
Denville, NJ 07834–2995
800-367-6274 New Jersey
201-625-7101
201-625-9053 TDD
> *Provides information to consumers on self-help groups and other organizations. Produces materials on how to establish a self-help group. Also publishes a directory of self-help and mutual-aid organizations.*

Office of Minority Health
Resource Center
1010 Wayne Ave., Suite 300
Silver Spring, MD 20910
800-444-6472
9:00 A.M. to 5:00 P.M. (eastern time), Monday to Friday
> *Provides information to minority groups on health topics that are of special interest to them. Information packet available upon request. English- and Spanish-speaking personnel available to callers.*

Office on Smoking and Health Hotline
Centers for Disease Control and Prevention
4770 Buford Hwy., NE, Mailstop K-50
Atlanta, GA 30341–3724
800-CDC-1311 (800-232-1311)
770-488-5705
> *Provides information on the health effects of smoking and materials relating to smoking-cessation programs.*

People's Medical Society
462 Walnut St., Lower Level
Allentown, PA 18102
800-624-8773
8:30 A.M. to 5:00 P.M. (eastern time), Monday to Friday
Answering machine at all other times
e-mail: Peoplesmed@Compuserve.com
> *Provides information on how to become a better-informed medical consumer. Also publishes consumer-oriented medical information on topics ranging from pediatrics to Medicare. Membership information and publications catalog available upon request.*

HEARING IMPAIRMENTS

American Speech-Language-Hearing Association Helpline
10801 Rockville Pike
Rockville, MD 20852
800-638-8255 Voice and TDD
800-897-8682 Alaska, Hawaii and Maryland
301-897-8682
e-mail: IRC@asha.org
8:30 A.M. to 4:30 P.M. (eastern time), Monday to Friday
> *Provides general information on speech, language and hearing problems. Also makes referrals to practitioners in the caller's area. Information packet available upon request.*

Better Hearing Institute
P.O. Box 1840
Washington, DC 20013
800-943-2746
703-642-0580
9:00 A.M. to 5:00 P.M. (eastern time), Monday to Friday
Answering machine at all other times
e-mail: Betterhearing@juno.com
> *Provides information on deafness and other types of hearing problems.*

Captioned Films for the Deaf
5000 Park St., N
St. Petersburg, FL 33709
800-237-6213 Voice and TDD
813-545-8781
8:00 A.M. to 5:00 P.M. (eastern time), Monday to Friday

Provides information on films with captioning that are available for persons with hearing impairments.

Deafness Research Foundation
9 E. 38th St., 7th Floor
New York, NY 10016–0003
800-535-3323 Voice and TTY
212-684-6556 New York City
9:00 A.M. to 5:00 P.M. (eastern time), Monday to Friday

Provides information on hearing problems. Makes referrals to physicians in the caller's area. Also provides information on how to select a hearing aid and detect hearing problems in children. Information packet available upon request.

Delta Society
P.O. Box 1080
Renton, WA 98057–1080
800-869-6898
206-226-7357
9:00 A.M. to 5:00 P.M. (Pacific time), Monday to Friday

Provides information on how to obtain hearing dogs for persons with hearing impairments.

Hear Now
4001 S. Magnolia Way, Suite 100
Denver, CO 80237
800-648-4327 Voice and TDD
303-758-4919 Colorado
8:30 A.M. to 4:00 P.M. (mountain time), Monday to Friday
Answering machine at all other times

Provides information on hearing aids and cochlear implants. Sponsors a national hearing aid bank. Also makes referrals to organizations and agencies in the caller's area.

Hearing Aid Hotline
20361 Middlebelt Rd.
Livonia, MI 48152
800-521-5247
313-478-2610

Provides information on hearing loss and hearing aids. Also makes referrals to hearing aid specialists in the caller's area.

Hearing Information Center
P.O. Box 1880
Media, PA 19063
800-622-3277
> *Provides hearing screening over the phone and answers general questions about hearing.*

National Captioning Institute
5203 Leesburg Pike
Falls Church, VA 22041
800-533-9673
703-998-2443
9:00 A.M. to 5:30 P.M. (eastern time), Monday to Friday
Answering machine at all other times
> *Provides captioning services for television programs and films. Information packet available upon request.*

**National Institute on Deafness and
Other Communications Disorders**
U.S. Department of Health and Human Services
National Institutes of Health Building
9000 Rockville Pike
Bethesda, MD 20892
800-241-1044
800-241-1055 TDD
301-402-0900
8:30 A.M. to 5:30 P.M. (eastern time), Monday to Friday
> *Provides information on resources that are available to hearing-impaired individuals and their families. Information packet available upon request.*

Sensor Hearing Aids
300 S. Chester Rd.
Swarthmore, PA 19081
800-622-3277
215-544-2700
9:00 A.M. to 5:00 P.M. (eastern time), Monday to Friday
> *Provides information on hearing loss and hearing aids. Also makes referrals to practitioners in the caller's area.*

TRIPOD Grapevine
2901 N. Keystone St.
Burbank, CA 91504
800-352-8888 Voice and TDD
800 287-4763 Voice and TDD California
9:00 A.M. to 5:00 P.M. (Pacific time), Monday to Friday
> *Provides information and services to parents who are raising hearing-impaired children.*

HEART DISEASE

American Heart Association
7272 Greenville Ave.
Dallas, TX 75231
800-242-8721
8:30 A.M. to 4:30 P.M. (central time), Monday to Friday
Provides information on coronary conditions. Also makes referrals to support groups in the caller's area.

Coronary Club
9500 Euclid Ave.
Cleveland, OH 44195
800-478-4255
216-444-3690
8:00 A.M. to 4:00 P.M. (eastern time), Monday to Friday
Answering machine at all other times
Provides information on heart care and rehabilitation, including surgery, medication, diet and exercise. Also provides information on the latest research involving the detection and treatment of heart disease.

National Society for MVP and Dysautonomia
880 Montclaire Rd., #280
Birmingham, AL 35213
800-541-8602
205-597-5765
8:15 A.M. to 4:30 P.M. (central time), Monday to Friday
Provides information on the diagnosis and treatment of mitral valve prolapse syndrome and dysautonomia. Also makes referrals to support groups in the caller's area.

HOSPICE

Children's Hospice International
900 N. Washington St., Suite 700
Alexandria, VA 22314
800-242-4453
703-684-0330 Virginia
8:30 A.M. to 5:30 P.M. (eastern time), Monday to Friday
Answering machine at all other times
Provides information on hospice programs especially designed for children with life-threatening conditions or who are terminally ill.

Hospice Education Institute
5 Essex Square
P.O. Box 713
Essex, CT 06246
800-544-2213
203-767-1620 Alaska and Connecticut
9:00 A.M. to 4:30 P.M. (eastern time), Monday to Friday
> *Provides information and counseling on death and dying and the role of the hospice. Publishes a national directory of hospice programs. Also makes referrals to agencies in the caller's area.*

National Hospice Organization
1901 N. Moore St., Suite 901
Arlington, VA 22209
800-658-8898
8:30 A.M. to 5:30 P.M. (eastern time), Monday to Friday
> *Provides information on hospice programs available in the caller's area.*

HOSPITAL CARE

Hill-Burton Hospital Program
Division of Facilities Compliance
Parklawn Building, Room 11-25
5600 Fishers Ln.
Rockville, MD 20857
800-638-0742
800-492-0359 Maryland
9:30 A.M. to 5:30 P.M. (eastern time), Monday to Friday
Answering machine at all other times
> *Provides information on hospitals that are participating in the Hill-Burton Free Care Program in the caller's area. Information packet available upon request.*

HUNTINGTON'S DISEASE

Huntington's Disease Society of America
140 W. 22nd St., 6th Floor
New York, NY 10011–2420
800-345-4372
212-242-1968
9:00 A.M. to 5:00 P.M. (eastern time), Monday to Friday
e-mail: curehd@hdsa.ttisms.com
> *Provides information and referrals to individuals with Huntington's disease and their families. Also offers crisis intervention and makes referrals to support groups in the caller's area. Information packet available upon request.*

IMMUNE DEFICIENCY DISEASES

Immune Deficiency Foundation
Courthouse Square
25 W. Chesapeake Ave., Suite 206
Towson, MD 21204
800-296-4433
9:00 A.M. to 5:00 P.M. (eastern time), Monday to Friday
Answering machine at all other times
> *Provides information to individuals and families affected by primary immune deficiency diseases. Also publishes educational materials and guidelines on starting support groups in the caller's area.*

INCONTINENCE

Help for Incontinent People (HIP)
P.O. Box 544
Union, SC 29379
800-252-3337
803-579-7902
8:00 A.M. to 5:00 P.M. (eastern time), Monday to Friday
Answering machine at all other times
> *Provides information on incontinence, including latest treatments and developments relating to assistive devices. Also offers suggestions on how to deal with incontinence.*

Simon Foundation for Continence
P.O. Box 815
Wilmette, IL 60091
800-237-4666
708-864-3913 Illinois
9:00 A.M. to 6:00 P.M. (central time), seven days a week
> *Provides information on incontinence. Also makes referrals to practitioners and support groups in the caller's area.*

INSURANCE

Alternative Health Insurance Services
P.O. Box 9178
Calabasas, CA 91372–9178
800-331-2713
818-509-5742 Los Angeles
> *Provides information on insurance plans that cover alternative health-care practitioners.*

Communicating for Seniors
P.O. Box 677
Fergus Falls, MN 56538
800-432-3276
218-739-3241
8:00 A.M. to 4:30 P.M. (central time), Monday to Friday
> *Provides information on insurance matters to older Americans,
> especially on Medicare supplemental insurance. Information packet
> available upon request.*

Co-op-America
2100 M St., NW, Suite 403
Washington, DC 20037
800-424-2667
202-872-5200 District of Columbia
> *Provides information on worker-owned and cooperatively structured
> health insurance plans that provide coverage for conventional as well
> as alternative practitioners.*

National Insurance Consumer Helpline
American Council of Life Insurance
Health Insurance Association of America
Insurance Information Institute
1001 Pennsylvania Ave., NW
Washington, DC 20004
800-942-4242
> *Provides general information on how to choose an insurance agent
> or broker and an insurance company. Also provides information on
> the following types of insurance: health, long-term-care, disability,
> Medicare supplemental and major medical. Does not provide
> information on specific policies or companies.*

KIDNEY DISEASES

American Association of Kidney Patients
100 S. Ashley Dr., Suite 280
Tampa, FL 33602
800-749-2257
813-251-0725 Tampa
9:00 A.M. to 5:00 P.M. (eastern time), Monday to Friday
> *Provides information to kidney patients and their families on how to
> cope with kidney diseases.*

American Kidney Fund
6110 Executive Blvd., Suite 1010
Rockville, MD 20852
800-638-8299
800-492-8361 Maryland
8:00 A.M. to 5:00 P.M. (eastern time), Monday to Friday
> *Provides information on kidney diseases and organ donor programs. Also offers financial assistance to kidney patients. Information packet available upon request.*

National Kidney Foundation
30 E. 33rd St.
New York, NY 10016
800-622-9010
8:30 A.M. to 5:30 P.M. (eastern time), Monday to Friday
> *Provides information on the latest research into kidney and urinary tract diseases, organ donations and transplant programs. Also provides materials for public education programs.*

National Medical Care Patient Travel Service
Reservoir Pl.
1601 Trapelo Rd.
Waltham, MA 02154
800-634-6254
> *Provides information to dialysis patients on how to arrange for dialysis at a National Medical Center dialysis facility while on vacation.*

PRK Foundation (polycystic kidney disease)
4901 Main St., Suite 320
Kansas City, MO 64112
800-753-2873
816-931-2600
9:00 A.M. to 5:00 P.M. (central time), Monday to Friday
Answering machine at all other times
e-mail: 75713.2275@Compuserve.com
> *Provides information on polycystic kidney disease. Also provides support to individuals and their families, raises money for research, publishes a newsletter and sponsors an annual conference.*

LEUKODYSTROPHY

United Leukodystrophy Foundation
2304 Highland Dr.
Sycamore, IL 60178
800-728-5483
815-895-3211
24 hours a day, seven days a week
e-mail: ULF@ceet.niu.edu
> *Provides information on leukodystrophy. Also provides information to caregivers and makes referrals to support groups in the caller's area.*

LIVER DISEASES

American Liver Foundation
1425 Pompton Ave.
Cedar Grove, NJ 07009
800-223-0179
201-857-2626 New Jersey
8:30 A.M. to 4:30 P.M. (eastern time), Monday to Friday
> *Provides information and assistance to children and adults with liver diseases. Also makes referrals to practitioners and support groups in the caller's area.*

Wilson's Disease
P.O. Box 75325
Washington, DC 20013
800-399-0266
703-636-3003
24 hours a day, seven days a week
> *Provides aid and mutual support to individuals and their families affected by Wilson's disease. Promotes research into discovering a treatment and cure for this condition.*

LIVING WILLS/ADVANCE DIRECTIVES

Choice in Dying
200 Varick St.
New York, NY 10014
800-989-WILL (800-989-9455)
212-366-5540
> *Provides information to persons interested in executing living wills or advance directives. Information packet available upon request.*

National Hemlock Society
P.O. Box 101810
Denver, CO 80250–1810
800-247-7421
> *Provides information on the rights of patients to make treatment decisions by executing advance directives.*

LUPUS

Lupus Foundation of America
4 Research Pl., Suite 180
Rockville, MD 20850–3226
800-558-0121
301-670-9292 Maryland
24 hours a day, seven days a week
> *Provides information on books written by doctors and patients who have lupus. Also makes referrals to chapters in the caller's area.*

Terri Gothelf Lupus Research Institute
3 Duke Pl.
South Norwalk, CT 06854
800-825-8787
203-852-0120
9:00 A.M. to 7:30 P.M. (eastern time), Monday to Friday
> *Provides information on medical centers that conduct research into the causes and treatment of lupus. Also provides general information on lupus to patients and their families. Information packet available upon request.*

LYME DISEASE

Lyme Disease Foundation
1 Financial Plaza, 18th Floor
Hartford, CT 06103
800-886-LYME (800-866-5963)
860-525-2000
24 hours a day, seven days a week
> *Provides information on the diagnosis, treatment and prevention of Lyme disease.*

LYMPHEDEMA

National Lymphedema Network
2211 Post St., Suite 404
San Francisco, CA 94115–3427
800-541-3259
24 hours a day, seven days a week
e-mail: lymphnet@hooked.net
> *Provides information on lymphedema to patients and their families. Information packet available upon request.*

MARFAN SYNDROME

National Marfan Foundation
382 Main St.
Port Washington, NY 11050
800-862-7326
8:30 A.M. to 3:30 P.M. (eastern time), Monday to Friday
Answering machine at all other times
e-mail: staff@marfan.org
> *Provides information to individuals who have Marfan syndrome and their families. Also maintains a support network for families, publishes a newsletter and holds conferences.*

McCUNE-ALBRIGHT SYNDROME

McCune-Albright Syndrome Division
Magic Foundation
1327 N. Harlem Ave.
Oak Park, IL 60302
800-362-4423
708-383-0808
9:00 A.M. to 5:00 P.M. (central time), Monday to Friday
e-mail: magic@nettap.com
> *Provides information and support to families of McCune-Albright patients. Also publishes a newsletter with medical information and makes referrals to support groups in the caller's area.*

MEDIC ALERT

Medic Alert Foundation International
2323 N. Colorado Ave.
Turlock, CA 95380
800-432-5378
800-468-1020 California
209-668-3333 Alaska and Hawaii
24 hours a day, seven days a week

> *Provides information on how to register with Medic Alert and obtain an emergency identification bracelet. The foundation also maintains a copy of the patient's medical record, which can be retrieved and sent to a practitioner or medical facility in the event of an emergency. Free registration form and catalog available upon request.*

MEDICARE/MEDICAID

Inspector General's Hotline
U.S. Department of Health and Human Services
P.O. Box 17303
Baltimore, MD 21203–7303
800-447-8477
800-638-3986 Maryland
800-269-0271 Social Security issues

> *Handles complaints from recipients relating to overcharges and possible fraud and waste of funds in the Medicare and Medicaid programs.*

Medicare Information Hotline
U.S. Department of Health and Human Services
Health Care Financing Administration
Washington, DC 20201
800-638-6833
8:00 A.M. to midnight, seven days a week

> *Provides general information on the Medicare program and responds to specific questions concerning Medicare coverage. Also provides information on Medicare supplemental insurance polices. Investigates complaints received from beneficiaries concerning alleged instances of supplemental insurance fraud or abuse.*

MEN'S HEALTH

American Prostate Society
1340 Charwood Rd., Suite F
Hanover, MD 21076
800-678-1238
410-850-0818
9:00 A.M. to 5 P.M. (eastern time), Monday to Friday
> *Provides information on prostate disease and works to increase public awareness. Information packet available upon request.*

Impotence Information Center
P.O. Box 9
Minneapolis, MN 55440
800-843-4315
8:00 A.M. to 5:30 P.M. (central time), Monday to Friday
Answering machine at all other times
> *Provides information on the causes and treatments of impotence but does not provide counseling. Also makes referrals to practitioners in the caller's area.*

Star Center
27211 Lahser Rd., Suite 208
Southfield, MI 48034
800-835-7667
313-357-1314 Michigan
24 hours a day, seven days a week
> *Provides general information on impotency. Also makes referrals to practitioners in the caller's area.*

Us Too (Prostate Cancer)
American Foundation for Urologic Disease
300 W. Pratt St., Suite 401
Baltimore, MD 21201
800-828-7866
> *Provides information on the latest developments in the diagnosis and treatment of prostate cancer. Also makes referrals to chapters in the caller's area.*

MÉNIÈRE'S DISEASE

Ménière's Network
Ear Foundation at Baptist Hospital
2000 Church St., Box 111
Nashville, TN 37236
800-545-4327 Extension 304 for TDD
615-329-7807 Voice and TDD
24 hours a day, seven days a week
  *Provides information on the diagnosis and treatment of
  Ménière's disease.*

MENTAL HEALTH

American Board of Professional Psychology
2100 E. Broadway, Suite 313
Columbia, MO 65201–6082
800-255-7792
  Provides information on certified psychologists in the caller's area.

American Mental Health Counselors Association
801 N. Fairfax St., Suite 304
Alexandria, VA 22314
800-326-2642
703-823-9800
8:30 A.M. to 4:30 P.M. (eastern time), Monday to Friday
  *Provides information on professionals in the counseling field.
  Also makes referrals to practitioners in the caller's area.*

American Mental Health Fund
1021 Price St.
Alexandria, VA 22314
800-433-5959
703-684-2201 Virginia
24 hours a day, seven days a week
  *Provides general information on mental illness. Also makes referrals to
  chapters in the caller's area. Information packet available upon request.*

American Schizophrenic Association
900 N. Federal Hwy., Suite 330
Boca Raton, FL 33432
800-847-3802
24 hours a day, seven days a week
  *Provides general information and educational materials about mental
  illnesses and learning disabilities. Also makes referrals to practitioners
  in the caller's area. Information packet available upon request.*

Camelback Helpline
7575 E. Earl Dr.
Scottsdale, AZ 85251
800-253-1334
24 hours a day, seven days a week

> *Provides information on subjects such as mental health, eating disorders and substance dependency. Also makes referrals to treatment centers in the caller's area. Information packet available upon request.*

Depression/Awareness, Recognition and Treatment Program (D/ART)
National Institute of Mental Health
Inquiries Branch
5600 Fishers Ln.
Rockville, MD 20857
800-421-4211 Spanish available
24 hours a day, seven days a week

> *Provides information on the causes, treatment and prevention of depression and related mental disorders.*

Knowledge Exchange Network (KEN)
National Mental Health Services
P.O. Box 42490
Washington, DC 20001
800-789-2647
301-984-6283
8:30 A.M. to 5:00 P.M. (eastern time), Monday to Friday

> *Provides information on mental health and resources available to families of those affected by mental health problems. Information packet available upon request.*

National Alliance for the Mentally Ill
2101 Wilson Blvd., Suite 302
Arlington, VA 22201
800-950-6264
9:00 A.M. to 5:00 P.M. (eastern time), Monday to Friday
Answering machine at all other times

> *Provides information on chapters, advocacy and support groups in the caller's area. Information packet available upon request.*

National Foundation for Depressive Illness
P.O. Box 2257
New York, NY 10116
800-248-4344
24 hours a day, seven days a week

> *Provides general information on depression. Also makes referrals to practitioners in the caller's area. Information packet available upon request.*

National Mental Health Association
1021 Prince St.
Alexandria, VA 22314–2971
800-969-6642
703-684-7722 Virginia
9:00 A.M. to 6:00 P.M. (eastern time), Monday to Friday

Provides information on mental health and mental illnesses. Also makes referrals to support groups, mental health centers, self-help clearinghouses and other organizations in the caller's area. Information packet available upon request.

MENTAL RETARDATION

American Association on Mental Retardation
444 N. Capital St., NW, Suite 846
Washington, DC 20001–1512
800-424-3688
202-387-1968
9:00 A.M. to 5:00 P.M. (eastern time), Monday to Friday
Answering machine at all other times
e-mail: aamr@access.digex.net

Provides general information on mental retardation. Also makes referrals to practitioners in the caller's area. Information packet available upon request.

MULTIPLE SCLEROSIS

Multiple Sclerosis Association of America
601-05 White Horse Pike
Oaklyn, NJ 08107
800-833-4672
9:00 A.M. to 5:00 P.M. (eastern time), Monday to Friday
Answering machine at all other times

Provides information and support to individuals affected by multiple sclerosis. Publishes a newsletter. Also makes referrals to support groups in the caller's area.

Multiple Sclerosis Foundation
6350 N. Andrew Ave.
Ft. Lauderdale, FL 33309
800-441-7055
305-776-6805
9:00 A.M. to 5:00 P.M. (eastern time), Monday to Friday
e-mail: MSFACTS@icanect.net
> *Provides information on the latest research into the cause, prevention, treatment and cure of multiple sclerosis. Works to improve the quality of life of people with multiple sclerosis. Also makes referrals to support groups in the caller's area.*

MYASTHENIA GRAVIS

Myasthenia Gravis Foundation
53 W. Jackson Blvd., Suite 660
Chicago, IL 60604
800-541-5454
8:00 A.M. to 5:00 P.M. (central time), Monday to Friday
> *Provides information on the diagnosis and treatment of myasthenia gravis. Also makes referrals to support groups in the caller's area.*

NEUROFIBROMATOSIS

Neurofibromatosis
8855 Annapolis Rd., Suite 110
Lanham, MD 20706–2924
800-942-6825
301-577-8984
24 hours a day, seven days a week
> *Provides information to individuals and families affected by neurofibromatosis. Makes referrals to support groups in the caller's area. Publishes a newsletter and promotes networking among families. Also assists in starting support groups.*

NUTRITION INFORMATION

Akpharma Foods
P.O. Box 111
Pleasantville, NJ 08232–0111
800-257-8650
9:00 A.M. to 5:00 P.M. (eastern time), Monday to Friday
> *Provides information on Beano, a product that helps people digest beans and vegetable fiber. Information packet and samples of the product available upon request.*

American Dietetic Association
Consumer Nutrition Hotline
216 W. Jackson Blvd., Suite 800
Chicago, IL 60606
800-366-1655
10:00 A.M. to 5:00 P.M. (central time), Monday to Friday
> *Provides general information on nutrition, including cholesterol,*
> *weight control and healthy snacks. Also makes referrals to nutritional*
> *counselors in the caller's area. Provides special service for teenagers.*

Beech-Nut Nutrition
Checkerboard Square
Consumer Affairs, 1-B
St. Louis, MO 63164
800-523-6633
800-492-2384 Pennsylvania
9:00 A.M. to 8:00 P.M. (eastern time), Monday to Friday
> *Provides information on the nutritional content of baby food and*
> *answers food-related questions.*

Garlic Information Center
Cornell Medical Center
800-330-8922
> *Provides information on the use of garlic as a seasoning and*
> *medicinal product.*

Gerber Hotline
Consumer Relations Gerber Products
445 State St.
Fremont, MI 49413
800-443-7237
24 hours a day, seven days a week
> *Provides information on infant nutrition and specific baby-care topics.*

HCF Foundation
High Carbohydrate Fiber
University of Kentucky
800 Rose St.
Lexington, KY 40536
800-727-4423
> *Provides information on the role of dietary fiber in regard to*
> *cholesterol, diabetes and blood sugar levels. Callers may leave*
> *specific questions on the voice-mail system.*

International Olive Oil Council

P.O. Box 2506
Stuart, FL 34995–2506
800-232-6548
9:00 A.M. to 5:00 P.M. (eastern time), Monday to Friday
Provides information on the nutritional and fat content of olive oil. Information packet available upon request.

Lactaid

McNeil Consumer Affairs
P.O. Box 85
Camp Hill Road
Ft. Washington, PA 19034
800-522-8243
9:00 A.M. to 5:00 P.M. (eastern time), Monday to Friday
Provides information on lactose intolerance and Lactaid, a product that assists in the digestion of lactose. Information packet and samples available upon request.

Meat and Poultry Hotline

U.S. Department of Agriculture
Room 1165 S, FSIS
Washington, DC 20250
800-535-4555
202-720-3333 District of Columbia
10:00 A.M. to 4:00 P.M. (eastern time), Monday to Friday
Provides information on the proper handling and storage of meat and poultry products. Information packet available upon request.

Molly McButter Information Hotline

800-622-3274
9:00 A.M. to 5:00 P.M. (eastern time), Monday to Friday
Provides information on the fat and calorie content of foods. Callers may speak directly with registered dietitians.

Mrs. Dash Sodium Information Hotline

800-622-3274
9:00 A.M. to 5:00 P.M. (eastern time), Monday to Friday
Provides low-sodium recipes and information on the sodium content of foods for people on sodium-restricted diets. Information packet available upon request.

Nutrition Hotline
American Institute for Cancer Research
1759 R St., NW
Washington, DC 20009
800-843-8114
202-328-7744 District of Columbia
9:00 A.M. to 9:00 P.M. (eastern time), Monday to Thursday
9:00 A.M. to 5:00 P.M. (eastern time), Friday
Answering machine at all other times
> *Provides information on the role of diet and nutrition in cancer*
> *prevention and how nutrition may be used to assist a cancer treatment*
> *program. Also responds to specific requests for information.*

Seafood Hotline
U.S. Department of Health and Human Services
Food and Drug Administration
Rockville, MD 20857
800-FDA-4010 (800-332-4010)
202-205-4314 District of Columbia
10:00 A.M. to 2:00 P.M. (eastern time), Monday to Friday
Answering machine at all other times
> *Provides information on how to buy and use seafood products.*
> *Callers may speak directly to food specialists or access prerecorded*
> *information on the proper handling and storage of seafood. List of*
> *seafood publications from the Food and Drug Administration*
> *available upon request.*

ORGAN DONOR PROGRAMS

The Living Bank
P.O. Box 6725
Houston, TX 77265
800-528-2971
713-528-2971
24 hours a day, seven days a week
> *Operates a registry and referral program for people wishing to donate*
> *their vital organs or bodies to research.*

National Marrow Donor Program
3433 Broadway St., NE, Suite 400
Minneapolis, MN 55413–1762
800-654-1247 Extension 149 for Spanish
8:00 A.M. to 6:00 P.M. (central time), Monday to Friday
Answering machine at all other times
> *Provides information on how to become a bone marrow donor.*

Organ Donor Hotline
United Network for Organ Sharing
1100 Boulders Pkwy., Suite 500
P.O. Box 13770
Richmond, VA 23225–8770
800-355-7527
804-330-8602
9:00 A.M. to 5:00 P.M. (eastern time), Monday to Friday
Answering machine at all other times
> *Provides information on organ donor programs and transplants. Also provides organ donor cards upon request.*

Transplant Recipients International Organization (TRIO)
1000 16th St., NW, Suite 602
Washington, DC 20036–5705
800-874-6386
9:00 A.M. to 5:00 P.M. (eastern time), Monday to Friday
Answering machine at all other times
e-mail: trio@primenet.com
> *Provides information and peer support to transplant recipients and their families. Conducts public education programs on the importance of organ donation. Also makes referrals to chapters in the caller's area.*

ORPHAN DRUGS AND RARE DISEASES

Friends of Karen
P.O. Box 190
Purdys, NY 10578
800-637-2774
9:00 A.M. to 5:00 P.M. (eastern time), Monday to Friday
> *Provides information on financial support that may be available to families with children who have rare or life-threatening diseases. Also provides information on support groups. Information packet available upon request.*

National Information Center for Orphan Drugs and Rare Diseases
P.O. Box 1133
Washington, DC 20013
800-336-4797
202-429-9091 District of Columbia
9:00 A.M. to 5:00 P.M. (eastern time), Monday to Friday
e-mail: nhicinfo@health.org
> *Provides information on how to locate a source for orphan drugs. (Orphan drugs, for which there is only a small market, are used to treat rare illnesses.)*

National Information Clearinghouse for Infants
  With Disabilities and Life-Threatening Conditions
University of South Carolina
Benson Building, 1st Floor
Columbia, SC 29208
800-922-9234 Voice and TDD
800-922-1107 Voice and TDD South Carolina
9:00 A.M. to 5:00 P.M. (eastern time), Monday to Friday
Answering machine at all other times

Provides information to families with children who have rare or life-threatening conditions. Also makes referrals to professional and community services in the caller's area. Offers special services to Vietnam veterans and their families.

National Organization for Rare Disorders
P.O. Box 8923
New Fairfield, CT 06812–1783
800-447-6673
800-833-8134 TDD
9:00 A.M. to 5:00 P.M. (eastern time), Monday to Friday
Answering machine at all other times

Provides information on how to apply for the drug cost-sharing program sponsored by the pharmaceutical industry. Information packet available upon request.

OSTEOPOROSIS

National Osteoporosis Foundation
1150 17th St., NW, Suite 500
Washington, DC 20036–4603
800-223-9994
202-223-2226

Provides information on osteoporosis, including a publication answering basic questions about the condition. Information packet available upon request.

OSTOMY

United Ostomy Association
36 Executive Park, #120
Irvine, CA 92714–6744
800-826-0826
714-660-8624
7:00 A.M. to 4:00 P.M. (Pacific time), Monday to Friday
Answering machine at all other times
> *Provides information on ostomy procedures and helps those with ostomies to lead normal lives. Also makes referrals to support groups in the caller's area. Information packet available upon request.*

OVER-THE-COUNTER MEDICATIONS

> *The following manufacturers of over-the-counter medications may be contacted for more information on the proper use of their products. Information lines are available 24 hours a day unless otherwise indicated.*

3M Personal Health Care
Building 515-3N-02
St. Paul, MN 55144–1000
800-537-2191

American Lifeline
103 S. Second St.
Madison, WI 53704
800-257-5433

AML Laboratories
1753 Cloverfield Blvd.
Santa Monica, CA 90404
800-800-1200

Astra USA
50 Otis St.
Westborough, MA 01581–4500
800-262-0460

Bausch & Lomb
Personal Products Division
1400 N. Goodman St.
P.O. Box 450
Rochester, NY 14692–0450
800-553-5340

Bayer Corporation
Consumer Care Division
36 Columbia Rd.
Morristown, NJ 07960–4518
800-331-4536

Blaine Company
1465 Jamike Ln.
Erlanger, KY 41018
800-633-9353

Blairex Laboratories
3240 N. Indianapolis Rd.
P.O. Box 2127
Columbus, IN 47202–2127
800-252-4739

Boiron
6 Campus Blvd., Building A
Newtown Square, PA 19073
800-258-8823

Bristol-Myers Products
345 Park Ave.
New York, NY 10154
800-468-7746

Care-Tech Laboratories
3224 S. Kingshighway Blvd.
St. Louis, MO 63139
800-325-9681

Church & Dwight Company
469 N. Harrison St.
Princeton, NJ 08543–5297
800-228-5635

Efcon Laboratories
P.O. Box 7499
Marietta, GA 30065–1499
800-722-2428

Iyata Pharmaceutical
735 N. Water St., Suite 612
Milwaukee, WI 53202
800-809-7918

Kyolic
Division of Wakunaga of America Company
23501 Madero St.
Mission Viejo, CA 92691
800-421-2998

Lederle Consumer Health
A Division of Whitehall-Robins Healthcare
5 Giralda Farms
Madison, NJ 07940–0821
800-282-8805

Marlyn Nutraceuticals
14851 N. Scottsdale Rd.
Scottsdale, AZ 85254
800-462-7596

McNeil Consumer Products
Division of McNeil-PPC
1 Campus Dr.
Somerset, NJ 08873
800-523-6225

Muro Pharmaceutical
890 East St.
Tewksbury, MA 01876–1496
800-225-0974

Ohm Laboratories
P.O. Box 7397
North Brunswick, NJ 08902
800-527-6481

Pfizer Pharmaceuticals
Consumer Health Care Group
Division of Pfizer
235 E. 42nd St.
New York, NY 10017–5755
800-723-7529

Pharmaton Natural Health Products
A Division of Boehringer Ingelheim Pharmaceutical
900 Ridgebury Rd.
Ridgefield, CT 06877
800-243-0127

Procter & Gamble
P.O. Box 5516
Cincinnati, OH 45201
800-358-8707

Requa
P.O. Box 4008
1 Senneca Pl.
Greenwich, CT 06830
800-321-1085

Roberts Pharmaceutical Corporation
4 Industrial Way, W
Eatontown, NJ 07724
800-828-2088

Ross Products Division
Abbott Laboratories
Columbus, OH 43215–1724
800-227-5767

Similasan Corporation
1321 S. Central Ave.
Kent, WA 98032
800-426-1644

SmithKline Beecham Consumer Healthcare
Unit of SmithKline Beecham
P.O. Box 1467
Pittsburgh, PA 15230
800-245-1040

Stellar Pharmacal Corporation
1990 N.W. 44th St.
Pompano Beach, FL 33064–8712
800-845-7827

Triton Consumer Products
561 E. Golf Rd.
Arlington Heights, IL 60005
800-942-2009

Wallace Laboratories
P.O. Box 1001
Half Acre Road
Cranbury, NJ 08512
800-526-3840

Warner-Lambert Consumer Helpline
Warner-Lambert Company
Consumer Health Products Group
201 Tabor Rd.
Morris Plains, NJ 07950
800-524-2854
800-223-0182

Whitehall-Robins Healthcare
American Home Products Corporation
5 Giralda Farms
Madison, NJ 07940–0871
800-322-3129
800-762-4672

PARALYSIS AND
SPINAL CORD INJURY

APA Spinal Cord Injury Hotline
2200 Kernane Dr.
Baltimore, MD 21207
800-526-3456
9:00 A.M. to 5:00 P.M. (eastern time), Monday to Friday
Answering machine at all other times
e-mail: SCIHOTLINE@aol.com

> *Provides information on spinal cord injuries. Also makes referrals to organizations, agencies and treatment centers in the caller's area.*

American Paralysis Association
Montebello Hospital
500 Morris Ave.
Springfield, NJ 07081
800-225-0292
201-379-2690 New Jersey
9:00 A.M. to 5:00 P.M. (eastern time), Monday to Friday
e-mail: Paralysis@aol.com

> *Provides information on the latest research into the treatment of spinal cord injuries and prospects for recovery. Information packet available upon request.*

National Spinal Cord Injury Association
8300 Colesville Rd., Suite 551
Silver Spring, MD 20910
800-962-9629
9:00 A.M. to 5:00 P.M. (eastern time), Monday to Friday
e-mail: NSCI2@aol.com
> *Provides information to patients and their families on services available
> from organizations, agencies and support groups in the caller's area.
> Information packet available upon request.*

PARENTING

A Way Out
P.O. Box 277
New Paltz, NY 12561
800-292-9688
914-255-1907
24 hours a day, seven days a week
> *Provides assistance to parents who are considering abducting their
> children or who already have taken their children. Also has a network
> of nationwide mediators who can help resolve custody disputes
> between parents.*

Child Reach
155 Plan Way
Warwick, RI 02886
800-556-7918 Extension 216 for TDD
> *Provides information on how to become a sponsor to a child living in
> the Third World.*

National Association for Parents of the Visually Impaired
P.O. Box 317
Watertown, MA 02272–0317
800-562-6265
617-924-3434
9:00 A.M. to 5:00 P.M. (eastern time), Monday to Friday
> *Provides general information and counseling to families with visually
> impaired children.*

Parents Without Partners
8807 Colesville Rd.
Silver Spring, MD 20910
800-637-7974
301-588-9354 Maryland
9:00 A.M. to 5:00 P.M. (central time), Monday to Friday
> *Provides information on support groups for single parents.
> Information packet available upon request.*

Technical Assistance to Parent Programs Network
Federation for Children With Special Needs
95 Berkeley St., Suite 104
Boston, MA 02116
800-331-0688 Massachusetts
9:00 A.M. to 5:00 P.M. (eastern time), Monday to Friday

Provides information to parents with children who have special needs because of developmental disabilities, including information on special education laws. Offers training and workshops for parents of children with special needs. Also makes referrals to support groups in the caller's area.

Toughlove International
P.O. Box 1069
Doylestown, PA 18901
800-333-1069
215-348-7090 Pennsylvania

Serves as a support group for parents of teenage children with behavioral problems. Also makes referrals in both the United States and Canada.

PARKINSON'S DISEASE

American Parkinson's Disease Association
1250 Hylan Blvd.
Staten Island, NY 10305
800-223-2732 New York
719-981-8001
9:00 A.M. to 5:00 P.M. (eastern time), Monday to Friday
Answering machine at all other times

Provides brochures and information packets on medicines used to treat Parkinson's disease. Also offers counseling services and makes referrals to treatment centers in the caller's area.

National Parkinson's Foundation
1501 N.W. Ninth Ave.
Miami, FL 33136
800-327-4545
800-433-7022 Florida
305-547-6666 Miami
8:00 A.M. to 5:00 P.M. (eastern time), Monday to Friday
e-mail: mailbox@NPF.Med.miami.edu

Provides information on Parkinson's disease. Also makes referrals to practitioners in the caller's area.

Parkinson's Disease Foundation
William Black Medical Research Building
710 W. 168th St.
New York, NY 10032
800-457-6676
9:00 A.M. to 5:00 P.M. (eastern time), Monday to Friday
e-mail: PDFCPMC@aol.com

> *Provides information on patient care and rehabilitation, including lists of self-help groups and of clinics where treatment is available. Clinical specialists are available to answer questions from callers.*

PESTICIDES

National Pesticides Telecommunications Network
National Pesticides Information Clearinghouse
Oregon State University
333 Weniger Hall
Corvalis, OR 97332–6502
800-858-7378
541-737-1197 TDD
24 hours a day, seven days a week
e-mail: MILLERT@ACE.ORST.EDU

> *Provides information to the public and the medical profession on the hazards of pesticides.*

PHARMACEUTICAL MANUFACTURERS
(Free Medication Program)

> *The following companies provide free medicine for economically disadvantaged persons through patient-assistance programs. Most of these companies ask that patients meet certain income requirements. Check with the individual companies to learn the requirements and the process for submitting an application.*

Abbott Laboratories/Ross Laboratories
1 Abbott Park Rd.
Abbott Park, IL 60064–3500
800-922-3255
708-937-6100

Allergan Prescription Pharmaceuticals
2525 Dupont Dr.
P.O. Box 19534
Irvine, CA 92713–9534
800-347-4500 Extension 6219
714-752-4500

Amgen
1840 Deharilland Dr.
Thousand Oaks, CA 91320–1789
800-272-9376
805-447-1000

Bristol-Myers Squibb
Bristol-Myers U.S. Pharmaceutical Division
P.O. Box 4500
Princeton, NJ 08543–4500
800-736-0003
609-897-2000

Genentech
460 Point San Bruno Blvd.
South San Francisco, CA 94080
800-879-4747
415-225-1000

GlaxoWellcome
5 Moore Dr.
P.O. Box 13408
Research Triangle Park, NC 27709
800-452-9677
919-248-2100

Hoechst-Marion-Roussel
Routes 202-206
P.O. Box 2500
Somerville, NJ 08876–1258
800-776-4563
908-231-2000

Hoffman-La Roche
340 Kingsland St.
Nutley, NJ 07110
800-526-6367
201-235-5000

Pfizer Pharmaceuticals
235 E. 42nd St.
New York, NY 10017–5755
800-869-9979
212-573-2323

Sandoz Pharmaceuticals Corporation
59 Route 10
East Hanover, NJ 07936
800-937-6673
201-503-7500

PHYSICIAN CREDENTIALING

ABMS Certification Line
American Board of Medical Specialties
47 Perimeter Center, E, Suite 500
Atlanta, GA 30346
800-776-2378
9:00 A.M. to 6:00 P.M. (eastern time), Monday to Friday
*Provides information on the certification status of physicians, in-
cluding their specialties and years in which they were certified. Caller
should have physician's name and location ready before calling.*

American Osteopathic Association
Department of Certification
142 E. Ontario St.
Chicago, IL 60611
800-621-1773
312-280-5845
9:00 A.M. to 5:00 P.M. (central time), Monday to Friday
*Provides information on osteopathy as a healing art. Also verifies the
specialty board certification of osteopathic physicians.*

POISON CONTROL CENTERS

See also: **PESTICIDES** and **TOXIC SUBSTANCES**

Note: *The following poison control centers are certified by the*
American Association of Poison Control Centers (AAPCC),
*3201 New Mexico Ave., NW, Suite 310, Washington, DC 20016.
There may be other poison control centers in your area; however, these
are the only centers that meet AAPCC standards. Unless otherwise
indicated, the toll-free number is only available in the state, section of
the state or area code shown.* ***In the event of an emergency, contact
the nearest hospital serving your area.***

ALABAMA

Alabama Poison Center
408-A Paul Bryant Dr.
Tuscaloosa, AL 35401
800-462-0800
205-345-0600 Tuscaloosa

Regional Poison Center
Children's Hospital of Alabama
1600 Seventh Ave., S
Birmingham, AL 35233
800-292-6678
205-939-9201 Birmingham
205-933-4050 Birmingham

ARIZONA

Arizona Poison and Drug Information Center
University of Arizona
Arizona Health Science Center, Room 1156
1501 N. Campbell Ave.
Tucson, AZ 85724
800-362-0101
520-626-6016 Tucson

Samaritan Regional Poison Center
Good Samaritan Regional Medical Center
Ancillary-1
1111 E. McDowell Rd.
Phoenix, AZ 85006
602-253-3334 Phoenix

CALIFORNIA

Central California Regional Poison Control Center
Valley Children's Hospital
3151 N. Millbrook, IN31
Fresno, CA 93703
800-346-5922 Central California
209-445-1222 Fresno

Regional Poison Control Center
University of California-Davis Medical Center
2315 Stockton Blvd.
Sacramento, CA 95817
800-342-9293 Northern California
916-734-3692 Sacramento

San Diego Regional Poison Center
University of California San Diego Medical Center
200 W. Arbor Dr.
San Diego, CA 92103–8925
800-876-4766 Accessible in area code 619

COLORADO

Rocky Mountain Poison and Drug Center
8802 E. Ninth Ave.
Denver, CO 80220
800-332-3073 Colorado
303-629-1123 Denver
800-860-0620 Idaho
800-525-5042 Montana
800-446-6179 Las Vegas

CONNECTICUT

Connecticut Poison Control Center
University of Connecticut Health Center
263 Farmington Ave.
Farmington, CT 06030
800-343-2722
203-679-3056 Farmington

DISTRICT OF COLUMBIA

National Capitol Poison Center
3201 New Mexico Ave., NW, Suite 310
Washington, DC 20016
202-625-3333
202-362-8563 TTY

FLORIDA

Florida Poison Information Center-Jacksonville
University Medical Center
University of Florida Health Science Center-Jacksonville
655 W. Eighth St.
Jacksonville, FL 32009
800-282-3171
904-549-4480 Jacksonville

Florida Poison Information Center-Miami
University of Miami School of Medicine
Department of Pediatrics
P.O. Box 016960 (R-131)
Miami, FL 33101
800-282-3171

Florida Poison Information Center and
   Toxicology Resource Center
Tampa General Hospital
P.O. Box 1289
Tampa, FL 33601
800-282-3171
813-253-4444 Tampa

GEORGIA

Georgia Regional Poison Control Center
Grady Memorial Hospital
80 Butler St., SE
P.O. Box 26066
Atlanta, GA 30335
800-282-5846
404-616-9000 Atlanta

INDIANA

Indiana Poison Control Center
Methodist Hospital of Indiana
1701 N. Senate Blvd.
P.O. Box 1367
Indianapolis, IN 46206
800-382-9097 Northern Indiana, northern Ohio, central
   and southern Michigan
317-929-2323 Indianapolis

KENTUCKY

Kentucky Regional Poison Center
Kosair Children's Hospital
Medical Towers South, Suite 572
P.O. Box 35070
Louisville, KY 40232
800-722-5725
502-589-8222 Louisville and southern Indiana

LOUISIANA

Louisiana Drug and Poison Information Center
Northeast Louisiana University
Sugar Hall
Monroe, LA 71209
800-256-9822
318-362-5393 Monroe

MARYLAND

Maryland Poison Center
University of Maryland School of Pharmacy
20 N. Pine St.
Baltimore, MD 21201
800-492-2414 Maryland
410-528-7701 Baltimore

National Capitol Poison Center (DC suburbs only)
3201 New Mexico Ave., NW, Suite 310
Washington, DC 20016
202-625-3333
202-362-8563 TTY

MASSACHUSETTS

Massachusetts Poison Control System
300 Longwood Ave.
Boston, MA 02115
800-682-9211
617-232-2120 Boston

MICHIGAN

Poison Control Center
Children's Hospital of Michigan
Harper Professional Building
4160 John Rd., Suite 425
Detroit, MI 48201
313-745-5711 Detroit

MINNESOTA

Hennepin Regional Poison Center
Hennepin County Medical Center
701 Park Ave.
Minneapolis, MN 55415
612-347-3141 Minneapolis
612-337-7474 TDD
612-337-7387 Petline

Minnesota Regional Poison Center
8100 34th Ave., S
P.O. Box 1309
Minneapolis, MN 55440–1309
612-221-2113 Minneapolis

MISSOURI

Regional Poison Center
Cardinal Glennon Children's Hospital
1465 S. Grand Blvd.
St. Louis, MO 63104
800-366-8888 Also serves western Illinois, Missouri
    and Topeka, Kansas
314-772-5200 St. Louis

MONTANA

Rocky Mountain Poison and Drug Center
8802 E. Ninth Ave.
Denver, CO 80220
800-525-5042 Montana

NEBRASKA

The Poison Center
Children's Memorial Hospital
8301 Dodge St.
Omaha, NE 68114
800-955-9119 Nebraska and Wyoming
402-390-5555 Omaha

NEW JERSEY

New Jersey Poison Information and Education System
Newark Beth Israel Medical Center
201 Lyons Ave.
Newark, NJ 07112
800-962-1253

NEW MEXICO

New Mexico Poison and Drug Information Center
University of New Mexico, North Campus
Health Science Library, Room 125
Albuquerque, NM 87131
800-432-6866
505-843-2551 Albuquerque

NEW YORK

Central New York Poison Control Center
SUNY Health Science Center
750 E. Adams St.
Syracuse, NY 13203
800-252-5655
315-476-4766 Syracuse

Finger Lakes Regional Poison Center
University of Rochester Medical Center
601 Elmwood Ave.
Box 321, Room G-3275
Rochester, NY 14642
800-333-0542
716-275-5151 Rochester

Hudson Valley Regional Poison Center
Phelps Memorial Hospital Center
701 N. Broadway
North Tarrytown, NY 10591
800-336-6997
914-366-3030 North Tarrytown

Long Island Regional Poison Control Center
Winthrop University Hospital
259 First St.
Mineola, NY 11501
516-542-2323 Mineola
516-542-2324 Mineola
516-542-2325 Mineola
516-542-3813 Mineola

New York City Poison Control Center
New York City Department of Health
455 First Ave., Room 123
New York, NY 10016
212-340-4494
212-689-9014 TDD

NORTH CAROLINA

Carolinas Poison Center
1012 S. Kings Dr., Suite 206
P.O. Box 32861
Charlotte, NC 28232
800-848-6946
704-355-4000 Charlotte

NORTH DAKOTA

North Dakota Poison Information Center
MediCare Medical Center
720 Fourth St., N
Fargo, ND 58122
800-732-2200
701-234-5575 Fargo

OHIO

Central Ohio Poison Control Center
Children's Hospital
700 Children's Dr.
Columbus, OH 43205
800-682-7625
614-228-2272 TTY
614-228-1323 Columbus

Cincinnati Drug and Poison Information Center and
   Regional Poison Control Systems
P.O. Box 670144
Cincinnati, OH 45267
800-872-5111
513-558-5111 Cincinnati

OREGON

Oregon Poison Center
Oregon Health Sciences University
3181 S.W. Sam Jackson Park Rd., CB550
Portland, OR 97201
800-452-7165
503-494-8968 Portland

PENNSYLVANIA

Central Pennsylvania Poison Center
University Hospital
Milton S. Hershey Medical Center
University Drive
P.O. Box 850
Hershey, PA 17033
800-521-6110
717-531-8335 TDD

Pittsburgh Poison Center
3705 Fifth Ave.
Pittsburgh, PA 15213
412-681-6669 Pittsburgh

The Poison Control Center
3600 Sciences Center, Suite 220
Philadelphia, PA 19104
800-521-6110
215-386-2100 Philadelphia

RHODE ISLAND

Rhode Island Poison Center
593 Eddy St.
Providence, RI 02903
401-444-5727 Providence

TENNESSEE

Middle Tennessee Poison Center
The Center for Clinical Toxicology
Vanderbilt University Medical Center
1161 21st Ave., S
501 Oxford House
Nashville, TN 37232
800-288-9999 Accessible in area code 615

TEXAS

Central Texas Poison Center
Scott & White Memorial Hospital
2401 S. 31st St.
Temple, TX 76508
800-764-7661

North Texas Poison Center
Parkland Hospital
5201 Harry Hines Blvd.
P.O. Box 35926
Dallas, TX 75235
800-441-0040
800-764-7661

Southeast Texas Poison Center
University of Texas Medical Branch
301 University Ave.
Galveston, TX 77550
800-764-7661
409-765-1420 Galveston
713-654-1701 Houston

UTAH

Utah Poison Control Center
410 Chipeta Way, Suite 230
Salt Lake City, UT 84108
800-456-7707 Utah
801-581-2151 Salt Lake City

VIRGINIA

Blue Ridge Poison Center
Box 67, Blue Ridge
University of Virginia Medical Center
Charlottesville, VA 22901
800-451-1428 Central, northern and western Virginia
804-924-5543 Charlottesville

National Capitol Poison Center (northern Virginia only)
3201 New Mexico Ave., NW, Suite 310
Washington, DC 20016
202-625-3333
202-362-8563 TTY

WASHINGTON

Washington Poison Center
155 N.E. 100th St., Suite 400
Seattle, WA 98125
800-732-6985
800-572-0638 TDD
206-526-2121 Seattle
206-517-2394 Seattle

WEST VIRGINIA

West Virginia Poison Center
West Virginia University School of Pharmacy
3110 MacCorkle Ave., SE
Charleston, WV 25304
800-642-3625
304-348-4211 Charleston

WYOMING

The Poison Center
Children's Memorial Hospital
8301 Dodge St.
Omaha, NE 68114
800-955-9119 Nebraska and Wyoming

PREGNANCY SERVICES

Abortion Hotline
National Abortion Federation
1436 U St., NW
Washington, DC 20009
800-772-9100
202-667-5881 District of Columbia
9:30 A.M. to 5:30 P.M. (eastern time), Monday to Friday
> *Provides information on services available at clinics in the caller's area. Also provides information on state laws applicable to abortion services.*

American Academy of Husband-Coached Childbirth
P.O. Box 5224
Sherman Oaks, CA 91413–5224
800-422-4784
818-788-6662 Sherman Oaks
24 hours a day, seven days a week
> *Provides information on the Bradley method of childbirth. Also makes referrals to practitioners in the caller's area. Information packet, including a directory of instructors, available upon request.*

American Society for Psychoprophylaxis in Obstetrics/Lamaze
1200 19th St., NW, Suite 300
Washington, DC 20036
800-368-4404
202-857-1128 District of Columbia
9:00 A.M. to 5:00 P.M. (eastern time), Monday to Friday
e-mail: aspo@sba.com
> *Provides information on the Lamaze technique. Also makes referrals to chapters in the caller's area.*

Be Healthy: Positive Pregnancy and Parenting Fitness
51 Saltrock Rd.
Baltic, CT 06330
800-433-5523
203-822-8573 Connecticut
9:00 A.M. to 5:00 P.M. (eastern time), Monday to Friday
Answering machine at all other times
> *Provides information on pregnancy and parenting, including audio and visual aids. Information packet available upon request.*

Bethany Christian Services
901 Eastern Ave., NE
Grand Rapids, MI 49503
800-238-4269
8:00 A.M. to midnight (eastern time), Monday to Friday
e-mail: LL@Bethany.org
> *Provides pregnancy testing, counseling services and adoption services to women. Information packet available upon request.*

Birthright
686 N. Broad St.
Woodbury, NJ 08096
800-848-5683
609-848-1818 New Jersey
8:00 A.M. to 3:00 P.M. (eastern time), Monday to Friday
> *Provides confidential pregnancy counseling to adolescents and women who are homeless because of their pregnancy. Also provides maternity and baby clothes and support services such as medical and financial referrals.*

Depression After Delivery
P.O. Box 1282
Morrisville, PA 19067
800-944-4774
215-295-3994
24 hours a day, seven days a week
> *Provides information to women who are experiencing postpartum depression. Also makes referrals to telephone support networks in the caller's area. Guidelines for starting support groups available upon request.*

Edna Gladney Center Pregnancy Hotline
2300 Hemphill St.
Ft. Worth, TX 76110
800-452-3639
817-926-3304 Texas
8:00 A.M. to 9:00 P.M. (central time), Monday to Friday
> *Provides information on all the options of pregnancy, especially adoption. Provides residential services to women who are considering placing their babies for adoption.*

Emergency Contraception Hotline
American College of Obstetricians and Gynecologists
409 12th St., SW
P.O. Box 96920
Washington, DC 20090–6920
800-584-9911
202-638-5577

> *Provides information and counseling on the steps to be taken to prevent conception in an emergency situation.*

International Childbirth Education Association
P.O. Box 20048
Minneapolis, MN 55420
800-624-4934

> *Provides information on pregnancy, childbirth and other related infant health needs. Also operates a book center. Information packet and catalog available upon request.*

La Leche League International
P.O. Box 1209
9616 Minneapolis Ave.
Franklin Park, IL 60131–8209
800-525-3243
9:00 A.M. to 3:00 P.M. (central time), Monday to Friday
> *Provides information on breast-feeding.*

Planned Parenthood Federation of America
810 Seventh Ave.
New York, NY 10019
800-829-7732
8:30 A.M. to 5:00 P.M. (eastern time), Monday to Friday
> *Provides information on family planning matters, including the use of contraceptives. Also makes referrals to Planned Parenthood clinics in the caller's area.*

PREMENSTRUAL SYNDROME
(PMS)

PMS Access
P.O. Box 9326
Madison, WI 53715
800-222-4767
608-257-8682 Wisconsin
9:00 A.M. to 5:00 P.M. (central time), Monday to Friday
Answering machine at all other times
> *Provides information on all aspects of premenstrual syndrome. Also makes referrals to practitioners in the caller's area. Information packet available upon request.*

PRODUCT SAFETY

U.S. Consumer Product Safety Commission
5401 Westbard Ave.
Bethesda, MD 20207
800-638-CPSC (800-638-3772)
800-638-8270 TDD
800-492-8104 TDD Maryland
9:00 A.M. to 5:00 P.M. (eastern time), Monday to Friday
> *Provides information on how to report complaints of injuries caused by consumer products.*

PSEUDOTUMOR CEREBRI

Pseudotumor Cerebri Society
1319 Butternut St., #3
Syracuse, NY 13208
800-926-1230
9:00 A.M. to 5:00 P.M. (eastern time), Monday to Friday
> *Provides information on the diagnosis and treatment of this condition. Also makes referrals to support groups in the caller's area.*

RETINITIS PIGMENTOSA

National Retinitis Pigmentosa Foundation
Executive Plaza One, Suite 800
11350 McCormick Rd.
Hunt Valley, MD 21031–1014
800-683-5555
800-683-5551 TDD
410-225-9400 Maryland
8:30 A.M. to 5:00 P.M. (eastern time), Monday to Friday
Answering machine at all other times
> *Provides information on the latest developments in the treatment of retinitis pigmentosa and responds to questions from callers.*

Retinitis Pigmentosa International Fighting Blindness
P.O. Box 900
Woodland Hills, CA 91365
800-344-4877
24 hours a day, seven days a week
> *Provides information on retinitis pigmentosa and reports on the latest research into the diagnosis and treatment of this condition.*

REYE'S SYNDROME

National Reye's Syndrome Foundation
426 N. Lewis St.
P.O. Box 8292
Bryan, OH 43506
800-233-7393
800-231-7393 Ohio
24 hours a day, seven days a week
e-mail: REYESSYN@mail.bright.net

> *Provides information on the symptoms and treatment of Reye's syndrome. Also makes referrals to support groups in the caller's area.*

SARCOIDOSIS

National Sarcoidosis Foundation
St. Michael's Medical Center
268 Martin Luther King Blvd.
Mail Drop 73B
Newark, NJ 07102
800-223-6429
201-624-4703
24 hours a day, seven days a week

> *Provides information and support services to families affected by sarcoidosis. Works to increase public awareness of this condition and assists in establishing support groups.*

SCOLIOSIS

Scoliosis Association
P.O. Box 811705
Boca Raton, FL 33481–1705
800-800-0669
24 hours a day, seven days a week

> *Provides information on scoliosis. Works to establish support networks for children and parents affected by this spinal condition. Publishes a newsletter and guidelines for starting support groups in the caller's area.*

SENIOR CITIZENS' SERVICES

Alcohol Rehabilitation for the Elderly
Hopedale Medical Complex
P.O. Box 267
Hopedale, IL 61747
800-354-7089
800-344-0824 Illinois
24 hours a day, seven days a week
> *Provides information on treatment programs for people ages 50 and older. Also makes referrals to support groups in the caller's area.*

Life Extension Foundation
995 S.W. 24th St.
Fort Lauderdale, FL 33315
800-327-6110
e-mail: LEF@lef.org
> *Provides information on antiaging research. Information packet available upon request.*

Lighthouse National Center for Vision and Aging
111 E. 59th St.
New York, NY 10022
800-334-5497
212-808-0077
212-808-5544 TDD
9:00 A.M. to 5:00 P.M. (eastern time), Monday to Friday
> *Provides information to senior citizens who may be or are at risk for visual impairment. Also conducts public education programs designed for senior citizens.*

National Council on the Aging
409 Third St., SW, Suite 200
Washington, DC 20024
800-424-9046
202-479-1200 District of Columbia
9:00 A.M. to 5:00 P.M. (eastern time), Monday to Friday
e-mail: info@NCOA.org
> *Provides general information on the subject of aging. Also serves as a clearinghouse for other organizations that provide programs to the elderly. Information packet available upon request.*

National Eye Care Project Hotline
P.O. Box 429098
San Francisco, CA 94142–9098
800-222-3937
8:00 A.M. to 4:00 P.M. (Pacific time), Monday to Friday
e-mail: Tjuring@aao.org

> *Provides information on a program designed for people ages 65 or older who are considered economically disadvantaged. Eligibility is based on income and resources available to the person. Also makes referrals to practitioners in the caller's area.*

National Institute on Aging Information Center
P.O. Box 8057
Gaithersburg, MD 20898–8057
800-222-2225
8:30 A.M. to 5:00 P.M. (eastern time), Monday to Friday
Answering machine at all other times

> *Provides information on all aspects of aging, especially those relating to healthy aging. Also provides information on the latest research into the biomedical, social and behavioral aspects of aging.*

National Meals on Wheels Foundation
2675 44th St., SW, Suite 305
Grand Rapids, MI 49509
800-999-6262
616-531-9909
8:30 A.M. to 4:30 P.M. (central time), Monday to Friday

> *Provides information on the Meals on Wheels programs. Assists organizations in starting programs and recruiting volunteers. Information packet available upon request.*

SEXUALLY TRANSMITTED DISEASES

STD National Hotline
American Social Health Association
P.O. Box 13827
Research Triangle Park, NC 27709
800-227-8922
919-361-8400 North Carolina
8:00 A.M. to 11:00 P.M. (eastern time), Monday to Friday

> *Provides confidential information on sexually transmitted diseases. Also makes referrals to practitioners in the caller's area.*

SJÖGREN'S SYNDROME

National Sjögren's Syndrome Association
3201 W. Evans Dr.
Phoenix, AZ 85023
800-395-6772
602-516-0787
8:00 A.M. to 5:00 P.M. (mountain time), Monday to Friday
Answering machine at all other times
e-mail: NSSA@aol.com
> *Provides information on Sjögren's syndrome. Information packet, along with a list of publications, available upon request.*

Sjögren's Syndrome Foundation
333 N. Broadway
Jericho, NY 11753
800-475-6473
516-933-6365
9:00 A.M. to 5:00 P.M. (eastern time), Monday to Friday
Answering machine at all other times
> *Provides information and educational materials. Encourages research designed to discover the causes of this condition and the development of an effective treatment. Also makes referrals to support groups in the caller's area.*

SKIN DISORDERS

American Hair Loss Council
P.O. Box 809313
401 N. Michigan Ave., 22nd Floor
Chicago, IL 60606–9313
800-274-8717
312-321-5128
9:00 A.M. to 5:00 P.M. (central time), Monday to Friday
Answering machine at all other times
> *Provides information on the latest research into the treatment of baldness in men and women. Information packet available upon request.*

American Society for Dermatological Surgery
930 N. Meacham Rd.
Schaumburg, IL 60173
800-441-2737
9:00 A.M. to 5:00 P.M. (central time), Monday to Friday
Answering machine at all other times
> *Provides information on surgical procedures related to skin damage from the sun, disease or aging. Also makes referrals to practitioners in the caller's area. Information packet available upon request.*

National Psoriasis Foundation
6600 S.W. 92nd Ave., #300
Portland, OR 97223
800-248-0886
503-244-7404
8:00 A.M. to 5:00 P.M. (Pacific time), Monday to Friday
Answering machine at all other times
e-mail: 76135.2746@Compuserve.com
> *Provides information on psoriasis. Information packet available upon request.*

United Scleroderma Foundation
P.O. Box 399
Watsonville, CA 95077–0399
800-722-4673
8:00 A.M. to 5:00 P.M. (Pacific time), Monday to Friday
e-mail: outreach@scleroderma.com
> *Provides information on scleroderma and other related skin diseases. Also makes referrals to support groups in the caller's area.*

SOCIAL SECURITY

National Association of Social Security
  Claimants Representatives
6 Prospect St.
Midland Park, NJ 07432
800-431-2804
914-735-8812 New York (call collect)
> *Provides the names of attorneys who specialize in Social Security cases.*

Social Security Hotline
Social Security Administration
U.S. Department of Health and Human Services
6401 Security Blvd.
Baltimore, MD 21235
800-772-1213
7:00 A.M. to 7:00 P.M. (eastern time), Monday to Friday
Answering machine at all other times
> *Provides information on Social Security claims and general information concerning eligibility for the program.*

SPASMODIC TORTICOLLIS

National Spasmodic Torticollis Association
P.O. Box 476
Elm Grove, WI 53122–0476
800-487-8385
24 hours a day, seven days a week

> *Provides referrals to practitioners and support groups in the caller's area. Information packet available upon request.*

SPEECH IMPAIRMENTS

American Speech-Language-Hearing Association Helpline
10801 Rockville Pike
Rockville, MD 20852
800-638-8255 Voice and TDD
800-897-8682 Alaska, Hawaii and Maryland
301-897-8682
8:30 A.M. to 4:30 P.M. (eastern time), Monday to Friday
e-mail: IRC@asha.org

> *Provides general information on speech, hearing and language problems. Also makes referrals to professionals in the field of speech therapy in the caller's area. Information packet available upon request.*

AT&T National Special Needs Center
2001 Route 46, 3rd Floor
Parsippany, NJ 07054
800-872-3883
800-833-3232 TDD
8:30 A.M. to 6:30 P.M. (eastern time), Monday to Friday

> *Provides information on purchasing or renting special equipment and services available to people with hearing, speech, vision or motion impairment.*

Institute of Logopedics
2400 Jardine Dr.
Wichita, KS 67219
800-835-1043 Includes Canada
800-937-4644 Canada
8:00 A.M. to 5:00 P.M. (central time), Monday to Friday

> *Provides information on services offered by the institute's outpatient audiology department.*

National Center for Stuttering
200 E. 33rd St., Suite 17-C
New York, NY 10016
800-221-2483
9:30 A.M. to 6:00 P.M. (eastern time), Monday to Friday
e-mail: executivedirector@stuttering.com

> *Provides information on methods used to treat stuttering in children and adults. Information packet available upon request.*

Stuttering Foundation of America
P.O. Box 11749
Memphis, TN 38111
800-992-9392
9:00 A.M. to 5:00 P.M. (central time), Monday to Friday
Answering machine at all other times

> *Provides information on stuttering to the public and works to assist speech pathologists in the treatment and prevention of stuttering. Also makes referrals to practitioners in the caller's area. Information packet available upon request.*

Stuttering Resource Foundation
123 Oxford Rd.
New Rochelle, NY 10804
800-232-4773
914-632-3925
24 hours a day, seven days a week

> *Provides information on stuttering. Also makes referrals in the caller's area to speech therapists who are specialists in treating stuttering disorders. Information packet available upon request.*

SPORTS MEDICINE

International Institute of Sports Science and Medicine
Center for Hip and Knee Surgery
1199 Hadley Rd.
Mooresville, IN 46158
800-237-7678 Indiana

> *Provides information on surgical procedures to repair hip and knee injuries.*

Women's Sports Foundation
Eisenhower Park
East Meadow, NY 11554
800-227-3988
9:00 A.M. to 5:00 P.M. (eastern time), Monday to Friday
e-mail: wosport@aol.com

> *Provides information on women and sports, physical fitness and sports medicine. Information packet available upon request.*

STROKE

AHA Stroke Connection
American Heart Association
7272 Greenville Ave.
Dallas, TX 75231
800-553-6321
214-373-6300
7:30 A.M. to 7:00 P.M. (central time), Monday to Friday
Answering machine at all other times
e-mail: strokaha@amhrt.org
> *Provides information on the diagnosis, treatment and prevention of stroke. Also makes referrals to support groups in the caller's area.*

National Aphasia Association
P.O. Box 1887
Murray Hill Station
New York, NY 10156–0611
800-922-4622
24 hours a day, seven days a week
> *Provides information materials to patients and their families. Also works to raise public awareness and makes referrals to support groups in the caller's area. Information packet available upon request.*

National Stroke Association
96 Inverness Dr., E, Suite 1
Englewood, CO 80112
800-787-6537
8:00 A.M. to 4:30 P.M. (mountain time), Monday to Friday
> *Provides information on support networks for stroke victims and their families. Also serves as a clearinghouse of information on stroke, including referrals to support groups in the caller's area.*

SUBSTANCE ABUSE: ALCOHOL AND DRUGS

Al-Anon Family Group Headquarters
1600 Corporate Landing Pkwy.
Virginia Beach, VA 23454
800-356-9996
800-344-2666 Meeting information line
800-443-4525 Canada
9:00 A.M. to 5:00 P.M. (eastern time), Monday to Friday
> *Provides information on 12-step recovery programs for alcoholics and their families. Information packet available upon request.*

Alcohol and Drug Referral Helpline
Highland Ridge Hospital
4578 S. Highland Dr.
Salt Lake City, UT 84117
800-821-4357
24 hours a day, seven days a week
Provides information on alcohol and drug abuse. Also makes referrals to support groups in the caller's area.

Alcohol Helpline
Adcare Hospital of Worcester
5 Northampton St.
Worcester, MA 01605
800-252-6465
24 hours a day, seven days a week
Provides basic information on alcohol treatment programs. Also makes referrals to treatment facilities in the caller's area.

Alcoholism and Drug Addiction Treatment Center
Scripps-Memorial Hospital
9904 Genesee Ave.
LaJolla, CA 92037
800-382-4357 California
619-457-4123
Provides information on substance abuse treatment programs. Also makes referrals to treatment services for adults and adolescents.

American Council for Drug Education
164 W. 74th St.
New York, NY 10023
800-488-3784
800-262-2463 Cocaine hotline
212-595-5810
24 hours a day, seven days a week
Provides information and referrals to drug rehabilitation programs in the caller's area. Also answers specific questions on substance abuse.

American Council on Alcoholism
2522 St. Paul St.
Baltimore, MD 21218
800-527-5344
410-889-0100 Baltimore
9:00 A.M. to 5:00 P.M. (eastern time), Monday to Friday
Answering machine at all other times
Provides information on alcoholism prevention programs for adults and children. Also provides counseling and referrals to treatment programs in the caller's area.

ASAP Treatment Hotline
P.O. Box 6150
Malibu, CA 90264
800-367-2727

> *Provides counseling and information on substance abuse treatment programs in the caller's area. Information packet available upon request.*

BABES World
Beginning Alcohol and Addiction Basic Education Studies
33 E. Forest St.
Detroit, MI 48201
800-542-2237

> *Provides information on alcohol and drug prevention programs designed for children. Information packet available upon request.*

Cocaine Anonymous
3740 Overland Ave., Suite G
Los Angeles, CA 90034
800-347-8998
310-559-5833 Los Angeles
24 hours a day, seven days a week

> *Provides information on cocaine addiction and rehabilitation programs. Information packet available upon request.*

Cottage Program International
75 E. Fort Union Blvd.
Midvale, UT 84047
800-752-6100
24 hours a day, seven days a week

> *Provides information on substance abuse treatment programs for families. Also makes referrals to chapters in the caller's area. Information packet available upon request.*

Drug Abuse Information and Treatment Referral Line
National Institute on Drug Abuse
11426 Rockville Pike, Suite 410
Rockville, MD 20852
800-662-4357
800-662-9832 Spanish
800-228-0427 TDD
9:00 A.M. to 3:00 P.M. (eastern time), Monday to Friday
Noon to 3:00 P.M. (eastern time), Saturday and Sunday
Answering machine at all other times

> *Provides counseling and referral services to callers. Also provides general information on substance abuse and addiction. Information packet available upon request.*

Drug Abuse Resistance Education (DARE)
P.O. Box 512090
Los Angeles, CA 90051–0090
800-223-3273

> *Provides information on programs that teach people how to avoid using drugs and other harmful substances. Information packet available upon request.*

Families Anonymous
P.O. Box 3475
Culver City, CA 90231
800-736-9805
818-989-7841
e-mail: famanon@earthlink.net

> *Provides information for families with children who have substance abuse or behavioral problems. Also provides counseling for family members and friends.*

Family Talk About Drinking
Anheuser-Busch Company
Department of Consumer Awareness and Education
1 Busch Pl.
St. Louis, MO 63118
800-359-8255
9:00 A.M. to 5:00 P.M. (central time), Monday to Friday
Answering machine at all other times

> *Provides information to families on how to discuss alcohol use with young children and teenagers. Message also available in Spanish. Information packet available upon request.*

Hazelton Foundation
15251 Pleasant Valley Rd.
P.O. Box 176
Center City, MN 55012
800-328-9000
800-262-5010 Minnesota
7:00 A.M. to 6:00 P.M. (central time), Monday to Friday
Answering machine at all other times

> *Provides information on substance abuse treatment and rehabilitation programs. Operates a rehabilitation center. Also makes referrals to other organizations and resources in the caller's area. Information packet available upon request.*

Johnson Institute
7205 Ohms Ln., Suite 200
Minneapolis, MN 55439–2159
800-231-5165
800-247-0484 Minnesota
e-mail: info@Johnsoninstitute.com
> *Provides educational materials and information on community
> substance abuse prevention programs in the caller's area.*

Mothers Against Drunk Drivers (MADD)
511 E. John Carpenter Freeway, Suite 700
Irving, TX 75062
800-438-6233
24 hours a day, seven days a week
> *Provides information on programs designed to prevent drunk driving.
> Information packet available upon request.*

National Clearinghouse for Alcohol and Drug Information
11426-28 Rockville Pike, Suite 200
Rockville, MD 20852
800-729-6686
8:00 A.M. to 5:00 P.M. (eastern time), Monday to Friday
e-mail: info@health.org
> *Provides information and referrals to callers with questions about
> alcohol and drug treatment programs in the caller's area. Information
> packet available upon request.*

National Council on Alcoholism and Drug Dependence Hopeline
12 W. 21st St.
New York, NY 10010
800-622-2255
212-206-6770 New York City
24 hours a day, seven days a week
> *Provides information on rehabilitation programs. Also makes referrals
> to support groups in the caller's area. Information packet available
> upon request.*

National Parents Resources Institute for Drug Education
3610 Dekalb Technology Pkwy., Suite 105
Atlanta, GA 30340
800-853-7867
404-577-4500 Atlanta
e-mail: PRC@MINDSPRING.Com
> *Provides information on how to start community drug education
> programs for young people. Information packet available upon request.*

New Life (Women for Sobriety)
P.O. Box 618
Quakertown, PA 18951
800-333-1606
215-536-8026
> *Provides assistance to women alcoholics. Information packet available upon request.*

Pride Institute
101 Fifth Ave.
New York, NY 10003
800-547-7433
24 hours a day, seven days a week
> *Provides information for persons addicted to alcohol or drugs. Also makes referrals to treatment centers in the caller's area.*

SUDDEN INFANT DEATH SYNDROME

American Sudden Infant Death Syndrome Institute
6065 Roswell Rd., Suite 876
Atlanta, GA 30328
800-232-7437
800-847-7437 Georgia
8:00 A.M. to 5:00 P.M. (eastern time), Monday to Friday
Answering machine at all other times
e-mail: parent@sids.org
> *Provides information on the latest research into the causes of sudden infant death syndrome. Also provides counseling and makes referrals to support groups in the caller's area. Information packet available upon request.*

Sudden Infant Death Syndrome Alliance
1314 Bedford Ave., Suite 210
Baltimore, MD 21208
800-221-7437
9:00 A.M. to 5:00 P.M. (eastern time), Monday to Friday
Answering machine at all other times
> *Provides information to parents of young infants. Also offers counseling and support services to parents who have lost a child to sudden infant death syndrome. Information packet available upon request.*

SURGERY SERVICES

American Academy of Facial Plastic and Reconstructive Surgery
1110 Vermont Ave., NW, Suite 220
Washington, DC 20005
800-332-3223
800-532-3223 Canada
202-842-4500 District of Columbia
24 hours a day, seven days a week
> *Provides general information on plastic surgery. Also makes referrals to practitioners in the caller's area.*

American Association of Oral and Maxillofacial Surgeons
9700 Bryn Mawr Ave.
Rosemont, IL 60018
800-467-5268
8:30 A.M. to 5:00 P.M. (central time), Monday to Friday
Answering machine at all other times
> *Provides information on temporomandibular joint and other jaw disorders, as well as oral cancer. Also makes referrals to practitioners in the caller's area. Information packet available upon request.*

American Plastic Surgery Information
6707 First Ave., S
St. Petersburg, FL 33707
800-522-2222 Florida
> *Provides information on plastic and reconstructive surgery. Also makes referrals to practitioners in the caller's area. Information packet available upon request.*

American Society of Plastic and Reconstructive Surgeons
444 E. Algonquin Rd.
Arlington Heights, IL 60005
800-635-0635
8:30 A.M. to 4:30 P.M. (central time), Monday to Friday
Answering machine at all other times
> *Provides information on surgical procedures. Also makes referrals to practitioners in the caller's area and verifies credentials of plastic surgeons. Information packet available upon request.*

Plastic and Aesthetic Surgery Center
217 E. Chestnut St.
Louisville, KY 40202
800-327-3613
800-633-8923 Kentucky
24 hours a day, seven days a week
> *Provides information on various plastic surgery procedures, including cost estimates. Also makes referrals to practitioners in the caller's area.*

SYRINGOMYELIA

American Syringomyelia Alliance Project
P.O. Box 1586
Longview, TX 75606–1586
800-ASAP-282 (800-272-7282)
903-236-7079
24 hours a day, seven days a week
> *Provides information and support to patients and their families. Also makes referrals to support groups in the caller's area. Sponsors an annual conference.*

TOURETTE SYNDROME

Tourette Syndrome Association
42-40 Bell Blvd.
Bayside, NY 11361
800-237-0717
9:00 A.M. to 5:00 P.M. (eastern time), Monday to Friday
Answering machine at all other times
e-mail: tourette@ix.netcom.com
> *Provides information on Tourette syndrome to patients and their families. Also makes referrals to chapters in the caller's area.*

TOXIC SUBSTANCES

Asbestos Technical Information Service
P.O. Box 12194
Research Triangle Park, NC 27709
800-334-8571
9:00 A.M. to 5:00 P.M. (eastern time), Monday to Friday
> *Provides information on different types of asbestos and proper removal and disposal procedures. Also provides information on home tests for asbestos. Information packet available upon request.*

Chemical Manufacturers Association
1300 Wilson Blvd.
Arlington, VA 22209
800-262-8200
202-887-1315 District of Columbia
9:00 A.M. to 6:00 P.M. (eastern time), Monday to Friday
Answering machine at all other times
e-mail: chemtrec@mail.cmahq.com
> *Provides general information on the safe handling of chemicals. Also makes referrals to the manufacturers of specific chemical products who are responsible for providing more detailed information on the proper use of their products. Information packet available upon request.*

Emergency Planning and Community Right-to-Know Information Hotline
U.S. Environmental Protection Agency
401 M St., NW
Washington, DC 20460
800-535-0202
202-479-2449 District of Columbia
9:00 A.M. to 6:00 P.M. (eastern time), Monday to Friday
Answering machine at all other times
> *Provides information on the types of chemicals that are stored and used in the community and workplace. Also provides information on the requirements of the Emergency Planning and Community Right-to-Know Act of 1986.*

Environmental Defense Fund Hotline
1616 P St., NW
Washington, DC 20036
800-225-5333
202-387-3500 District of Columbia
9:00 A.M. to 5:00 P.M. (eastern time), Monday to Friday
> *Provides information to the public on the issue of environmental protection, including ways in which individuals can help keep the environment clean. Information packet available upon request.*

National Center for Toxicological Research
3900 NCTR Rd.
Jefferson, AR 72079–9502
800-638-3321
9:00 A.M. to 5:00 P.M. (central time), Monday to Friday
> *Provides information on the effects of toxic substances on the environment.*

TUBEROUS SCLEROSIS

National Tuberous Sclerosis Association
8181 Professional Pl., Suite 110
Landover, MD 20785
800-225-6872
301-459-9888 Maryland
9:00 A.M. to 5:00 P.M. (eastern time), Monday to Friday
Answering machine at all other times
e-mail: ntsa@aol.com

> *Provides referrals to representatives of the association. Also provides information on parent-to-parent support networks in the caller's area. Information packet available upon request.*

UROLOGIC DISEASES

American Foundation for Urologic Disease
300 W. Pratt St., Suite 401
Baltimore, MD 21201
800-242-2383
410-727-2908
8:00 A.M. to 10:00 P.M. (eastern time), Monday to Friday

> *Provides information on the various types of adult and pediatric urologic diseases. Promotes research and conducts education programs to raise the public awareness on these conditions. Sponsors the Us Too prostate cancer survivors program. Information packet available upon request.*

VIETNAM VETERANS

Vietnam Veterans Agent Orange Victims
P.O. Box 2465
Darien, CT 06820–0465
800-521-0198
9:00 A.M. to 4:00 P.M. (eastern time), Monday to Friday
Answering machine at all other times

> *Provides medical and legal advice, information and counseling to veterans who have been exposed to the defoliant Agent Orange. Operates a children's fund to aid families whose children may be suffering from birth defects and developmental disabilities linked to Agent Orange. Information packet available upon request.*

VISION IMPAIRMENTS

See also: **RETINITIS PIGMENTOSA**

American Council of the Blind
1155 15th St., NW, Suite 1155
Washington, DC 20005
800-424-8666
202-467-5081 District of Columbia
3:00 P.M. to 5:30 P.M. (eastern time), Monday to Friday
e-mail: ncrabb@access.digex.net
> *Provides information and referrals to clinics, organizations and government agencies that provide services to the blind. Information packet available upon request.*

American Foundation for the Blind
11 Pennsylvania Ave., Suite 300
New York, NY 10001
800-232-5463
212-502-7662 TDD
8:30 A.M. to 4:30 P.M. (eastern time), Monday to Friday
e-mail: afbinfo@abf.org
> *Provides answers to questions concerning vision loss and blindness. Information packet available upon request.*

American Printing House for the Blind
1839 Frankfort Ave.
P.O. Box 6085
Louisville, KY 40206–6085
800-223-1839
502-895-2405
> *Provides information on braille, large-type books and computer disks for visually impaired persons. Information packet and catalog available upon request.*

AT&T National Special Needs Center
2001 Route 46, 3rd Floor
Parsippany, NJ 07054
800-872-3883
800-833-3232 TDD
8:30 A.M. to 6:30 P.M. (eastern time), Monday to Friday
> *Provides information on purchasing or renting special equipment and services available to people with hearing, speech, vision or motion impairment.*

Audio Reader
P.O. Box 847
Lawrence, KS 66044
800-772-8898 Kansas
> *Provides information on reading services available to visually impaired persons.*

Blind Children's Center
4120 Marathon St.
Los Angeles, CA 90029–0159
800-222-3566
800-222-3567 California
e-mail: info@blindcntr.org
> *Provides information on blindness. Also makes referrals to organizations and support groups in the caller's area.*

Books on Tape
P.O. Box 7900
Newport Beach, CA 92658–7900
800-626-3333
> *Provides information on how to obtain books on tape for visually impaired persons. Information packet available upon request.*

Guide Dog Foundation for the Blind
371 E. Jericho Turnpike
Smithtown, NY 11787
800-548-4337
9:00 A.M. to 5:00 P.M. (eastern time), Monday to Friday
e-mail: guidedog@guidedog.org
> *Provides information on the guide dog program. Also makes referrals to support groups in the caller's area.*

Job Opportunities for the Blind
1800 Johnson St.
Baltimore, MD 21230
800-638-7518
12:30 P.M. to 5:00 P.M. (eastern time), Monday to Friday
> *Provides career counseling, job listings and referrals to visually impaired persons who are seeking employment.*

National Service for the Blind and Physically Handicapped
National Library of Congress
1291 Taylor St., NW
Washington, DC 20542
800-424-8567
202-794-8650 District of Columbia
8:00 A.M. to 4:30 P.M. (eastern time), Monday to Thursday
e-mail: nls@loc.gov
> *Provides information on libraries that offer books on audiotape and books in braille.*

National Society to Prevent Blindness
National Center for Sight
500 E. Remington Rd., Suite 200
Schaumburg, IL 60173
800-221-3004
8:00 A.M. to 5:00 P.M. (central time), Monday to Friday
e-mail: 7477.100@Compuserve.com
> *Provides literature on specific vision problems and conditions. Also produces educational materials and offers professional education programs. Information packet available upon request.*

Recording for the Blind
20 Roszel Rd.
Princeton, NJ 08540
800-221-4792
609-452-0606
9:00 A.M. to 9:00 P.M. (eastern time), Monday to Friday
Answering machine at all other times
> *Provides information on how to obtain recordings for visually impaired persons. Information packet available upon request.*

WOMEN'S HEALTH

See also: **PREGNANCY SERVICES;**
PREMENSTRUAL SYNDROME

Breast Implant Information Service
Food and Drug Administration
P.O. Box 1802
Rockville, MD 20704–1802
800-532-4440
800-688-6167 TDD
10:00 A.M. to 4:00 P.M. (eastern time), Monday to Friday
Answering machine at all other times
> *Provides information on the status of clinical studies being conducted on the safety of silicone-gel-filled breast implants. Information packet available upon request.*

DES Action
1615 Broadway, Suite 510
Oakland, CA 94612
800-337-9288
510-465-4011
> *Provides information on the effects of DES (diethylstilbestrol) on the children of mothers who took the medication while pregnant. Promotes public awareness and offers support to DES-affected daughters and sons. Information packet available upon request.*

Johnson and Johnson
Personal Products Consumer Response Center
New Brunswick, NJ 08901
800-526-3967

> *Provides information on a wide range of women's health concerns, including toxic shock syndrome.*

Planned Parenthood Federation of America
810 Seventh Ave.
New York, NY 10019
800-829-7732
8:30 A.M. to 5:00 P.M. (eastern time), Monday to Friday

> *Provides information on a wide range of women's health issues, including general health and wellness, family planning, patient education and abortion. Also makes referrals to Planned Parenthood clinics in the caller's area.*

Women's Sports Foundation
Eisenhower Park
East Meadow, NY 11554
800-227-3988
9:00 A.M. to 5:00 P.M. (eastern time), Monday to Friday
e-mail: wosport@aol.com

> *Provides information on women and sports, physical fitness and sports medicine. Information packet available upon request.*

INDEX AND
SUBJECT CROSS-REFERENCE

Braille *See* Vision Impairments
Breast Cancer *See* Cancer
Breast Implant Information *See* Women's Health
Bulimia *See* Eating Disorders
Burn Care 28

C

Cancer 29
Captioned Films *See* Vision Impairments
Cerebral Palsy *See* Birth-Related Disorders
Chemical Hazards *See* Toxic Substances
Child Abuse *See* Children's Services; Domestic Violence/
    Sexual Abuse; Parenting
Child Nutrition *See* Nutrition Information
Child Pornography *See* Children's Services; Domestic Violence/
    Sexual Abuse
Child Sexual Abuse *See* Children's Services; Domestic Violence/
    Sexual Abuse
Child Substance Abuse *See* Substance Abuse: Alcohol and Drugs
Childbirth *See* Pregnancy Services
Childhood Cancer *See* Cancer
Children's Services 34
Chronic Fatigue Syndrome 40
Cleft Palate *See* Birth-Related Disorders
Cocaine Abuse *See* Substance Abuse
Colitis *See* Digestive Diseases
Communication Systems *See* Disabled Persons' Services;
    Emergency Medical Communication Systems
Computer Systems *See* Disabled Persons' Services
Contraception *See* Women's Health
Cornelia de Lange Syndrome *See* Birth-Related Disorders
Cosmetic Surgery *See* Surgery Services
Craniofacial Deformities *See* Surgery Services
Crohn's Disease *See* Digestive Diseases
Cystic Fibrosis *See* Birth-Related Disorders
Cystinosis *See* Birth-Related Disorders

D

Deaf Children *See* Hearing Impairments
Deafness *See* Hearing Impairments
Dental Care 40
Depression *See* Mental Health

S

Sarcoidosis 99
Scoliosis 99
Schizophrenia *See* Mental Health
Scleroderma *See* Skin Disorders
Self-Help Groups *See* Health Information
Senior Citizens' Services 100
Sexual Abuse *See* Domestic Violence/Sexual Abuse; Parenting
Sexually Transmitted Diseases 101
Shriners Hospitals *See* Burn Care; Children's Services
Sickle Cell Anemia *See* Anemia
Single Parent Groups *See* Parenting
Sjögren's Syndrome 102
Skin Disorders 102
Social Security 103
Sodium Information *See* Nutrition Information
Spasmodic Torticollis 104
Speech Impairments 104
Speech Pathologists *See* Speech Impairments
Speech Problems *See* Speech Impairments
Spina Bifida *See* Birth-Related Disorders
Spinal Cord Injury *See* Paralysis and Spinal Cord Injury
Sports Medicine 105
Stroke 106
Sturge-Weber Syndrome *See* Birth-Related Disorders
Stuttering *See* Speech Impairments
Substance Abuse: Alcohol and Drugs 106
Sudden Infant Death Syndrome 111
Surgery Services 112
Syringomyelia 113

T

Talking Books *See* Vision Impairments
Tay-Sachs Disease *See* Birth-Related Disorders
Teen Suicide *See* Children's Services
Telecommunications Equipment *See* Emergency Medical
     Communication Systems; Disabled Persons' Services;
     Hearing Impairments; Speech Impairments;
     Vision Impairments
Terminal Illnesses *See* Children's Services; Hospice
Tourette Syndrome 113